What Every Pa...
—and Child—
Should Know

Long before a child reaches sexual maturity, she or he needs to learn about child sexual abuse, AIDS, STDs, and contraception. Unfortunately, all too often, many of today's kids know more about sex than their parents do. This leaves them no other option than to continue trusting the information they are receiving from their friends, information that often is not only inaccurate but dangerous.

Guiding a child's development and answering questions about sexual matters honestly and without embarrassment is not easy for many parents. *BEYOND THE BIRDS AND THE BEES* will help you to become more comfortable with the process. In addition, it will encourage you to take the initiative instead of waiting for your child to ask questions, and to use opportunities in everyday life to make it clear to your child that sexual issues are a normal part of our lives and can be talked about comfortably.

—*from* BEYOND THE BIRDS AND THE BEES

BEYOND THE BIRDS AND THE BEES:

Fostering Your Child's Healthy Sexual Development

Beverly Engel

POCKET BOOKS

New York London Toronto Sydney Tokyo Singapore

The author of this book is not a physician, and the ideas, procedures, and suggestions in this book are not intended as a substitute for the medical advice of a trained health professional. All matters regarding your health require medical supervision. Consult your physician before adopting the suggestions in this book, as well as about any condition that may require diagnosis or medical attention.

An *Original* Publication of POCKET BOOKS

POCKET BOOKS, a division of Simon & Schuster Inc.
1230 Avenue of the Americas, New York, NY 10020

Engel, Beverly.
    Beyond the birds and the bees : fostering your child's healthy
sexual development / Beverly Engel.
        p.   cm.
    Includes bibliographical references and index.
    ISBN: 0-671-53570-6
    1. Sex instruction.   2. Sex instruction for children.   3. Sex
instruction for teenagers.   I. Title.
HQ31.E743   1997
613.9'51—dc21   97-19252
                                                   CIP

First Pocket Books trade paperback printing December 1997

10 9 8 7 6 5 4 3 2 1

POCKET and colophon are registered trademarks of
Simon & Schuster Inc.

Cover design by Patrice Kaplan
Text design by Stanley S. Drate/Folio Graphics Co. Inc.

Printed in the U.S.A.

This book is dedicated to Dylan and Kyle.

Acknowledgments

I wish to acknowledge researchers in the field of sexuality such as David Finklehor, and Masters and Johnson; pioneering authors such as Dorothy Corkville Briggs; child development experts such as Berry Brazelton; and sex educators and experts such as Mary Calderone for their dedication and invaluable information.

I want to thank all my clients throughout the years, from whom I learned a great deal.

A special thanks to my agent, Nancy Love, who was excited about the project from the beginning, and to my editor, Claire Zion, and Dan Slater, who meticulously edited the book.

Contents

✦ PART II ✦

NORMAL STAGES OF SEXUAL DEVELOPMENT: WHAT TO EXPECT AND WHAT TO TELL YOUR CHILD

Introduction

As a sex therapist and marriage counselor with twenty-three years' experience, I have worked with hundreds of people suffering from all types of sexual conflicts, sexual dysfunction, sexual-identity confusion, lack of sexual desire, and numerous other sexual problems. I have counseled people who felt sex was so shameful they could not share a sexual relationship—not even with the one they love; who were so afraid of sex that their bodies had become numb to almost all sexual sensation; or who were so inhibited that they could not communicate about sex even with their partners of twenty or more years. Almost all of these problems were caused by early childhood experiences—negative parental messages regarding masturbation and other natural sexual responses; a lack of privacy and disregard for individual rights in the family; a negative body image; or sexual abuse by parents, other relatives, or older children.

While I was able to treat these clients successfully, I felt it was a shame that they had to spend so much of their time *undoing* their childhood and *unlearning* negative messages and inaccurate information about sex.

Most of us, in fact, while our experience has not been as extreme, have had to recover from some negative programming concerning sex and have had to work hard to reestablish a healthy relationship with our body and our sexual and sensual selves. But why should we have to spend so much time trying to recapture what was our birthright—our natural, spontaneous sexuality?

Children are not born ashamed of their sexual feelings or ashamed of their bodies. Nor are they born afraid of their sexuality or afraid to be touched. And children are not born distrustful and afraid of intimacy either. They get that way

1

because of the way they are raised and because of the society in which we live. For this reason, I decided to write a book to help parents raise their children in such a way as to encourage them to remain unashamed and spontaneous. I wanted to help parents raise children who feel good about their sexuality and good about their bodies; who have healthy attitudes about their sexual feelings and those of others; children who are free to experience the sight, sound, taste, smell, and touch of their own sensuality; children who can communicate sexually in a direct, open, honest, assertive, and spontaneous manner; children who respect themselves enough to practice healthy sexuality. I wanted to help parents avoid many of the mistakes their parents made in raising them.

I have also worked with married couples, single parents, divorced parents, and gay parents and have shared in their struggles to raise sexually healthy children. Through this experience I discovered that parents all too often pass on to their children the misinformation, negative messages, and unhealthy sexual behavior they received as children. And they pass on their sexual hang-ups, fears, and anxiety. Parents don't do this intentionally, of course. In fact, many of the parents I have worked with have tried desperately *not* to pass on their sexual problems to their children. But first they needed to work on their own unresolved sexual issues and conflicts, work through their sexual shame, and begin to look at their sexuality in a whole new light. Because of this I realized I would need to offer more than just information on how to raise a sexually healthy child, I must also offer parents the chance to become more sexually healthy themselves.

And so I address the issues of parents' sexuality, parents' sexual concerns, problems, and attitudes, and how these interfere with their being good role models and teachers for their children.

In addition, I know that parents are overwhelmed and confused by the current sexual climate. They are deeply concerned with how all the sexual messages that their children are bombarded with daily are affecting their children. How do you raise a child to have a healthy interest in sex, to look forward to an exciting, active sex life, when all they hear about is people dying of AIDS, teenage pregnancy, and sexually transmitted diseases (or STDs)?

Unhealthy sexual images are blatantly used to capture our attention and our money. Advertisers portray unhealthy sex to sell products. We are constantly being barraged by sexual messages that contradict the healthy messages we want our children to hear. But examples of healthy sex are harder to find.

In *Beyond the Birds and the Bees* I focus a great deal of attention on how parents can work to counteract the negative sexual messages all around us. I also give up-to-date information on exactly what is happening with our young people today and offer facts on everything from AIDS and STDs to current trends like sadomasochism and bisexuality so that parents will know exactly what they are dealing with.

There are numerous books on how to talk to your children about sex by experts on child development, many of which I strongly recommend. But *Beyond the Birds and the Bees* offers far more than advice on how to talk to children about sex. It offers a specific strategy for raising sexually healthy children, children who are self-confident, safe, and assertive, children who will grow up to be adults capable of having an intimate, sensuous relationship with someone they love.

There is another very important topic that other books on childhood sexuality do not address. That is the issue of body image. Body image affects a person's ability to have a healthy, rewarding sex life in very profound ways. If we feel physically attractive, we will undoubtedly have a lot more confidence in our sexuality and our sexual attractiveness. But we live in a culture that dictates that females must be beautiful to be worthwhile, and then sets up standards of female beauty that are not only impossible for most females to live up to, but are unhealthy as well. For example, getting and staying thin have become a major pastime for females, consuming a significant amount of their time, energy, and money.

Until very recently, male children have not had to suffer quite as much pressure regarding the way their bodies should look, but all that is rapidly changing. Today, males are constantly being pressured to work out, pump up their muscles, and stay physically fit. The message that male children get today is that all females prefer a male who is athletic and muscular.

If parents go along with these ways of thinking and place an inordinate amount of importance on physical attractiveness, they are setting their children up for future problems. If, on the other hand, they teach their children to appreciate and respect their bodies, to see there is no single standard for determining physical attractiveness, and to determine their own and others' attractiveness based on other factors in addition to physical attractiveness, they will be contributing greatly to their child's healthy sexual development.

Before we get started, let me tell you a little more about myself. As well as being a sex therapist and sex educator with twenty-three years' experience working with individuals, couples, and families, I am the author of seven books, many of which address the subject of sexual self-esteem and childhood sexual abuse. These include: *Raising Your Sexual Self-Esteem; The Right to Innocence: Healing the Trauma of Child Sexual Abuse; Partners in Recovery: How Mates, Lovers, and Other Pro-survivors Can Learn to Support and Cope with Adult Survivors of Childhood Sexual Abuse;* and *Families in Recovery: Working Together to Heal the Damage of Childhood Sexual Abuse.*

I have trained other professionals throughout the United States and Canada on how to work with victims of childhood sexual abuse, and I have been interviewed on many national television and radio programs, including Oprah Winfrey, Phil Donahue, and CNN.

I am a recognized expert in the field of sexuality, having specialized in sexual dysfunction, sexual-orientation confusion, sexual addiction, and sexual abuse. I have also done extensive research on the impact of touch, parental messages, body image, and childhood trauma on the development of children's sexuality and am also an expert in these areas. Most parents, and even many therapists, are out of touch with what is going on with kids today, but I have kept abreast of the current issues that concern children, adolescents, and young adults.

In addition, as a nationally recognized expert on child sexual abuse and date rape, I am able to offer parents valuable information on how they can protect their children and teach them to be safe and assertive, as well as help parents whose children have already been abused or raped. I can also help those parents who have themselves been sexually abused, raped, or sexually harassed and are concerned about passing on their fears and problems to their children.

Healthy sexuality is a wonderful gift you can give your child. Our sexuality can provide us great pleasure and relaxation, cause us to reach great heights of ecstasy, provide us a way of achieving great intimacy with another human being, and allow us to connect with ourselves both physically and emotionally.

Unfortunately, it can also cause us a great deal of distress, pain, frustration, and disappointment. Most of this distress and pain can be alleviated if children are raised to be sexually healthy. I sincerely hope this book will help you in your determination to raise a sexually healthy child.

Part I

RAISING
A SEXUALLY
HEALTHY CHILD

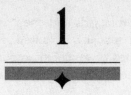

1

A Few Preliminary Words

Today's parents have more to worry about concerning their children than any other generation. They worry about their children's health, their safety, their education, and what kind of world they will have to face when they are grown. In spite of all they are distressed about, parents are now beginning to worry about another aspect of their child's life—their child's sexuality.

Being concerned about your child's sexuality is not necessarily a new phenomenon, but today's parents have far more to worry about than their parents and grandparents did. At one time in the not too distant past, parents felt they only needed to worry about two things concerning their child's sexuality—their daughter's getting pregnant or their son's being "trapped" into marriage by a pregnancy; and their child's contracting a venereal disease. Today, parents are not as naive about problems such as childhood sexual abuse and rape, and now they have much more dreaded venereal diseases to worry about, such as AIDS. And there are other concerns as well:

✦ In the United States, the average age for first intercourse is 16.2 for females and 15.7 for males. In the inner city, studies show this as low as 12.6 for females and 12.3 for males.

+ In 1992, one in four girls and one in six boys reported that they had been sexually assaulted. Recent studies report much higher rates of sexual intercourse among teens who have been abused, including higher rates of pregnancy and multiple partners.
+ Twenty-nine percent of all rapes occurred when the victims were younger than age eleven, with 61 percent of all reported rapes occurring before the victim reached age eighteen.
+ Of one hundred and sixty women treated for sexual dysfunction, it was found that 90 percent had been raped during childhood, 23 percent by fathers and stepfathers. Evidence confirms that molestation by a trusted caretaker is one of the most damaging forms of childhood sexual abuse.
+ At the college level, one in four women will be sexually assaulted during her four years at college. Seventy percent to 80 percent of those women will know their perpetrator. Nationally, the incidence of date rape is highest among women in their first year of college.
+ One man in fifteen will attempt to force sexual activity upon an acquaintance or date sometime during his four years at college.
+ Every year, two and a half million U.S. teenagers are infected with an STD (sexually transmitted disease).
+ Twenty percent of new AIDS cases are among young adults in their twenties. Given the virus's latency period, that means that most were infected in their teens.
+ The World Health Organization estimates that more than fourteen million adults and a million children are HIV-infected worldwide.

These are but some of the things parents today have to be worried about concerning their child's sexuality. There's more. Unhealthy sex is all around us: children starting to have sex at seven and eight years old . . . child pornography . . . pedophiles on the Internet . . . children having children . . . teenage prostitution . . . gay bashing . . . teachers having sex with their students . . . girls being sexually harassed in school . . . sex gangs where boys compete to see how many girls they can have sex with . . . teenage boys dating forty-year-old women . . . teens having sadomasochistic parties.

On top of all these problems, young people today are more confused about sex than ever before. They have more freedom, more information, and more options available to them concerning sex, but with this freedom comes the pressure of having to make choices, choices that even adults have difficulty making.

Sex has always been a confusing issue. But if sex was confusing for us when we were growing up, imagine how confusing it is for today's children. They are growing up in a time of extremes, a time when they are receiving conflicting messages about sex every day.

For example, sex is everywhere—on television, billboards, magazines, videos, and in the movies. Children and teenagers are bombarded with the message: "Sex is the most wonderful, exciting thing that can ever happen to you. It's a high better than any drug. It makes you powerful, mysterious, interesting, popular. Sexy girls get all the guys, and sexy guys get all the girls."

At the same time another message is being hammered into their heads daily: "Sex leads to AIDS, have sex and you risk dying." How in the world do we expect our children to come to terms with such blatantly conflicting messages?

And there are other conflicting messages. At the same time that there is a chastity movement encouraging teens to remain virgins until marriage, there is an equally powerful sexual revolt movement encouraging them to break all the rules and to experiment with multiple partners, sadomasochism, exhibitionism, voyeurism, etc.

Kids of today even get conflicting messages from their heros. Some popular icons like Madonna, Courtney Love, and R.E.M.'s Michael Stipe advocate experimenting with bisexuality, while several heavy metal bands advocate gay bashing.

In addition, today's children are exposed to all kinds of sexual activities and preferences, far more than their parents ever were. Few of us were exposed to such issues as transsexuality, sexual fetishes, and sadomasochism when we were growing up. But today's kids are exposed to these things daily just by turning on the television and watching one of the numerous daytime talk shows. Until recently, parents worried only about the messages their kids were receiving from hard rock and heavy metal bands concerning drugs and promiscuity. But today, in addition to drugs, kids are exposed to bondage and discipline, transvestitism, necrophilia, and misogyny by their favorite bands. While it can be argued that our society is in fact more progressive now, I think it is clear that children and teens are exposed to these various lifestyles prematurely and that it is bound to confuse them.

Kids of today are receiving other negative messages about sex as well. While many male rap stars advocate promiscuity, disrespect toward women, sexual harassment, and sexual brutality against women (rape, gang rape, sodomy), some female rap stars advocate promiscuity and using men sexually. Only a few rap stars try to balance it all out with messages about love and respect.

And even though we have entered a time when sex can be dangerous, it is also a time of new freedom concerning our sexuality in an entirely different way—in terms of sexual orientation and sexual preferences. Ironically, although sex has once again become risky, sexual practices that have in the past been considered forbidden are now in vogue, not only with teens but with adults. Practices such as sadomasochism, exhibitionism, and voyeurism have all become popular. Issues of ambiguity in sexual gender and orientation, such as in the cases of transsexualism, transvestitism, and bisexuality, are not only out of the closet, but in store windows and on television. And, at the same time, homosexuality has become the focus of debate as our country grapples with the complicated issues surrounding it in a way we never have before.

While the discussion around these issues is much needed, it nevertheless complicates an already difficult situation. Not only do we and our kids need to worry about sexually transmitted diseases, we and they now worry more about whether they are gay or straight, whether their propensity for voyeurism is normal or abnormal, and whether they (and we) should act out sexual fantasies. Sex has become more complicated than ever, and while we have more answers than before, we also have more conflicting answers.

In addition, the pressure seems to be on for both males and females not only to be physically perfect, but to be sexually superior. Kids today worry far more than we ever did about whether they are physically appealing or not, whether they are sexually exciting enough, and whether they can satisfy their lovers. Boys worry more about the state of their erections and how long they can last, while girls worry about whether they can have an orgasm and even if they can have multiple orgasms.

Whew! With all this, it's no wonder parents feel overwhelmed when it comes to raising a sexually healthy child. No wonder they feel lost when it comes to knowing what to do and which way to turn. Even the most educated, sophisticated, and experienced parents are plagued by questions like: How is it possible to raise a child who is safe from being exploited, molested, or raped? How is it possible to raise a child with healthy sexual values? And how is it possible to raise a child who will grow up to become a sexually healthy adult, one who is capable of enjoying a deep, meaningful relationship with someone he or she loves?

In spite of the fact that you are raising your child in such an unhealthy world, there is hope. As a parent you definitely will have more of an influence on your child than *any* other person or factor in your child's life. You can not only prepare her or him for the dangers and challenges of the world, but *counteract* the dangers, misinformation, and negative influences of others. You can provide your child with confidence, education, encouragement, and a positive body image—all essential building blocks to a healthy sexuality. You alone have the opportunity to give your child the gift of healthy sexuality.

How do you raise a child in such a world? More specifically, how do you raise a sexually healthy child in this kind of environment? The answer to this question is multi-leveled.

First of all, you as a parent need to educate yourself. This includes learning how you can best influence your child's sexuality in healthy ways, learning all you can about the sexual influences in your child's life, and learning what it means to be a child or teen in today's world.

You as a parent need to understand that what you don't know about sexuality today can hurt your children. You need to educate yourself about sexual practices and trends among young people that you are probably unaware of. You need to learn about sexual lifestyles and practices (such as voyeurism, exhibitionism, sadomasochism, and cross-dressing) that may not interest you or may even repulse you, in order to properly inform your children.

In our parents' day, the issue of sexuality was something that people just didn't talk about the way we do today. Our parents and grandparents were unfortunately a bit naive about sex and about their children's sexuality in particular. Today, parents are realizing that they can't afford to be unconcerned or naive about their child's sexuality.

Second, you will need to begin communicating with your child about sex at a very early age. You can't protect your child by trying to shield him or her from all the negative sexual messages that are being communicated to him or her. You need instead to educate your child and provide him or her with healthy values to counter the unhealthy ones he or she is receiving.

Long before a child reaches sexual maturity, she or he needs to learn about child sexual abuse, AIDS, STDs, and contraception. Unfortunately, all too often, many of today's kids know more about sex than their parents. This leaves them no other option than to continue trusting the information they are receiving from their friends, information that often is not only inaccurate but dangerous.

Guiding a child's development and answering questions

about sexual matters honestly and without embarrassment is not easy for many parents. *Beyond the Birds and the Bees* will help you to become more comfortable with the process. In addition, it will encourage you to take the initiative instead of waiting for your child to ask questions, and to use opportunities in everyday life to make it clear to your child that sexual issues are a normal part of our lives and can be talked about comfortably.

While it is difficult to know how much to teach children about sex, when to talk to them about it, and even how to tell them about it, talking to children about sex is only a small part of what this book is about.

Parents today need to know a whole lot more than how to talk to their children about sex. The changes in sexual behavior, attitudes, and lifestyles that have taken place in our society in the past few decades present today's parents and children with some of the most complex issues they will ever confront. It isn't enough for parents simply to tell their children about "the birds and the bees" anymore, or even to tell them they can feel free to ask any questions or talk anytime about sex. Nowadays, parents need to prepare their children not only for adulthood, but for the potential hazards of living in this time and the confusion they are bound to feel with all the sexual messages and options that are being presented to them.

Last, but certainly not least, in order to raise a sexually healthy child, parents must be sexually healthy themselves. Parents can do everything right in terms of raising their children, can know all they need to know about sex and pass on this information to their children in loving ways, but if they have unresolved sexual issues, conflicts, or sexual problems, those problems will be communicated to their children. Therefore, they need to work on their own sexual issues, whether it be a poor body image, sexual shame, sexual fears, or sexual dysfunction. In addition, parents need to explore their own sexual attitudes and beliefs and find a way to pass on those that will help their children grow into healthy adults and discard those that are false, unhealthy, too restrictive, or too permissive.

SEXUALLY HEALTHY PARENTS

A sexually healthy child comes from sexually healthy parents. What are the qualities of sexually healthy parents? Sexually healthy parents:

+ Desire for their children to grow into adults who are able to experience the joys, excitement, and fulfillment of sensuality and sexuality.

+ Recognize that it is what they don't know that will hurt their children and are dedicated to learning all they can about sex and the current sexual trends so they can pass the information on to their children.

+ Want to instill in their children positive values concerning sex, including the value of respecting other people's bodies, privacy, and personal limits.

+ Want to make certain that they do not pass on negative, non-life-affirming messages about sex, but instead teach their children positive esteem-enhancing messages.

+ Do not pass on negative or unhealthy information concerning sex, sex roles, gender differences, and so on, but strive to teach their children healthy, non-shame-inducing and nonexploitive attitudes about sex.

+ Are not weighed down by unexamined sexual guilt and shame from their own childhoods.

+ Are aware of their own sexual problems, hang-ups, and fears, understand where their problems originated, and are actively working on healing these past wounds as well as making an effort not to pass on these problems to their children.

+ Do not impose their own emotional or sexual needs onto their children.

+ Respect their children's need for privacy concerning their body and possessions, including their right to privacy in the bathroom and in their bedrooms.

✦ Are willing to discuss sex openly with their children and answer their questions about sex, and are able to admit to their children when they are uncomfortable.

✦ Are loving parents, capable of emotional and physical intimacy. Are comfortable showing affection to their mate and their children.

✦ Believe that sexual feelings are a normal part of life, even for children.

✦ Recognize that while children do not have the same kind of sexual feelings that adults do, they are in fact sexual and sensual beings.

✦ Recognize that while they cannot *protect* their children completely from the harsh realities of life, they can *prepare* their children for such realities.

✦ Recognize that while it is important to teach their values to their children, they must also respect their children's decisions and the independent choices they make in their lives.

WHAT IS A SEXUALLY HEALTHY CHILD?

Sometimes the best way to describe a sexually healthy child is to contrast him or her with a sexually unhealthy one. *A sexually unhealthy child:*

✦ Feels his or her genitals are shameful, dirty, or evil.

✦ Is uneducated about sex and the dangers of child molestation, rape, and date rape.

✦ Is full of shame about his or her sexual feelings.

✦ Has a poor body image, is overly critical of her or his body, believing that no boy or girl will like her or him because she or he is too fat, thin, short, tall, unattractive, or not "well-endowed" enough.

✦ Imposes his or her desires and will on younger children or on the opposite sex.

✦ Does not feel free to talk to his or her parents about sexual concerns or fears, or to ask questions about sex, genitals, sexual roles, etc.

✦ Feels she or he needs to hide sexual feelings and desires from her or his parents and other adults.

✦ Is so unhappy, troubled, or confused that she or he escapes into sexual fantasies or compulsive sexual behavior in order to relieve tension, anger, or pain, or to gain some comfort.

✦ Engages in sexual activities that are inappropriate for his or her age.

✦ Engages in sexual activities with other children as a way of feeling empowered or as a way of releasing anger.

✦ Is unable to say no to unwanted sexual advances by peers, older children, or adults.

Now let's contrast these qualities with those of a sexually healthy child. For example, among other things, *a sexually healthy child:*

✦ Knows the proper names of his or her genitals and considers them just another part of his or her body, albeit a private part.

✦ Has appropriate boundaries.

✦ Has a positive body image.

✦ Is aware of the dangers of child molestation and rape.

✦ Knows how to be assertive about letting people know when and under what circumstances she or he wants to be touched.

✦ Knows that sexual feelings are normal and healthy, but that we don't always have to act them out.

✦ Is in touch with his or her sensuality as well as his or her sexuality.

✦ Has impulse control.

A sexually healthy child is an educated child, one who has learned enough about healthy sexuality at home that she or he does not have to learn all about sex from friends and the media. Conversely, a sexually healthy child is one who has learned enough about *unhealthy* sexuality that he or she is not vulnerable to exploitation and manipulation by older children or adults, one who knows the difference between good touch and bad touch, and one who has learned what age-appropriate sexual behavior is.

A sexually healthy child is an assertive child, one who understands he or she has the right to privacy in the bathroom and bedroom, one who knows he or she has the right to say no and is able to do so, whether it is saying no to unwanted advances by a peer, an older child, or an adult. And it is a child who knows how to ask for help and keep asking until she or he gets it.

A sexually healthy child is one who feels free—to explore his or her body and to ask questions about sex and his or her body. It is one who does not feel ashamed of normal, healthy sexual feelings, one who is not burdened with negative messages regarding masturbation, his or her body, sexual feelings, sexual roles, or ideas about the opposite sex.

A sexually healthy child is an equitable child, one who respects the privacy and limits of others, one who does not try to impose her or his will on those younger or weaker, one who respects her or his body and the bodies of others.

And a sexually healthy child has a positive body image. He or she is not pressured (either externally or internally) to have a "perfect" body, but has been encouraged to love, respect, and appreciate his or her body for the wonderful gift it is.

Sexually healthy children grow up to be sexually healthy adults. They are less likely to be sexually abused or exploited, sexually harassed, or to become sexual at too early an age.

At this point, you may feel overwhelmed. You may be asking yourself, "How can I make certain I'm doing the right things to insure that my child will grow up sexually healthy? What if I make mistakes?

No one is talking about perfection here. This is where the book you are reading comes in. It will teach you how to raise a sexually healthy child instead of a sexually unhealthy one.

Step by step, I will take you through the most difficult situations you will face concerning your child's sexuality, including:

+ How to establish proper boundaries concerning your privacy and the privacy of your child.
+ How to deal with the issue of masturbation.
+ How and when to begin sex education.
+ How to teach children about potential dangers without frightening them.
+ How to teach children your values and beliefs without encouraging rebellion.

Fortunately, most parents today are smart enough to realize that sexuality is a major part of life and that being well-adjusted sexually is an important part of being an all-around well-adjusted, healthy human being. They are educated enough to realize that their child's sex education begins early on in life and is not confined to school programs, but occurs every day. And they are aware that their own early sexual experiences and education had a profound effect not only on their sexuality but on their body image and ability to trust, be vulnerable, and be intimate.

If you are reading this book it is because you are an exceptional parent, one who doesn't wish to put your head in the sand, one who wants the best for your child no matter how uncomfortable it might make you, and one who has learned from the mistakes your own parents made and who doesn't want to make the same mistakes.

Facing the issue of your child's sexuality is not an easy matter. Most parents would just as soon forget about this aspect of their child's life or at least postpone it until their child reaches puberty. But as we all know, children do not wait for their parents to get comfortable with an issue before they start experiencing problems with it. Your child has already started developing sexual attitudes, beliefs, and fears, and he or she isn't going to wait for you to get comfortable before developing more.

Your child needs you as a source of accurate information, as a healthy role model, as a confidant, and as a nurturer. As an infant, he or she needs you as the one who will introduce touching, bonding, intimacy, trust, and vulnerability. As a toddler, he or she needs you to be a healthy role model showing her or him, by your example, how loving couples interact, how touch is used to connect with others, to heal hurts, to soothe and comfort. As a young child, he or she needs you to answer questions and to provide accurate information on sexuality, his or her body, relationships, the opposite sex, and to do so in a comfortable, self-assured way instead of one that is couched in secrecy and shame. And as he or she enters puberty and all through adolescence, he or she needs you as a confidant, one he or she can feel comfortable coming to to talk about his or her concerns and problems regarding sexuality. All this will take a lot of work on your part, but it will be well worth it.

In order for you to fulfill all these roles for your child, you will need to work through many of your own sexual hang-ups and unfinished business.

At the end of each chapter is a section entitled "Parental Issues" in which I address personal issues that you as a parent may have concerning the topic of the chapter, the likely cause of your difficulties, and suggestions on how you can work on these issues. This will be followed by exercises designed to help you begin to overcome the problem or to elicit important information concerning your attitudes and beliefs about the topic.

This book will help you no matter what your circumstances or concerns. Some of you are worried about whether you can raise a sexually healthy child because you don't believe you received a healthy upbringing yourself. Those of you who had sexual concerns as a child and those who currently have sexual problems may fear you will pass these on to your child.

Some of you are currently worried about a particular aspect of your child's sexuality and have found nowhere else to turn. For example, those who have recently discovered their child engaging in sexual activities with other children will want to know just what kind of behavior is normal sex play and what is symptomatic of other problems.

And many parents feel overwhelmed with what they see and hear going on with teenagers today. These parents want a book that will explain the current trends and offer suggestions on how to discuss them with their children.

Beyond the Birds and the Bees will deal with all these issues as well as the concerns of parents who are just starting their families. I hope that you will refer to the book throughout your child's growing years. It is more than just a book about "how to talk to your child about sex." It is a strategies-oriented book on exactly how to go about raising your children in such a way as to encourage healthy attitudes about sex and their bodies.

The book is divided into two parts. Part I addresses what you as a parent need to do in order to raise a sexually healthy child. Part II is divided into the four major developmental stages of childhood sexuality—the preschool years (ages 2–5), the school years (ages 6–9), preadolescence (ages 10–12), and adolescence (ages 13–18)—and will address the issues that arise during each stage of development. In addition, I suggest topics that parents should bring up for each age period as well as list the most frequently asked questions from children at each stage with suggestions as to how to answer them. At the end of each of the four developmental chapters, there will once again be a section entitled "Parental Issues."

Also included in Part II are chapters on "Special Problems of Adolescence" such as teenage pregnancy, date rape, and the issue of teenage homosexuality.

The information in this book applies to all parents: married, separated, divorced, unmarried; heterosexual, homosexual, and bisexual. While there are obviously some differences between heterosexual and homosexual individuals and couples, these differences are far outweighed by the common desire to provide their children with the best education and example possible.

Today's parents are faced with problems that their parents never had to face and so are their children. Raising a sexually healthy child may seem to some an impossibility given all that is going on, but in fact it is not. While it is certainly difficult, it is still possible to raise a child who respects his or her own body and those of others, who has a healthy attitude about sex, viewing it neither as a shameful thing, a tool for exploitation, or a toy to play with. It is still possible to raise a child who will grow into sexual maturity looking forward to having a loving, pleasurable experience with someone she or he cares deeply about. *Beyond the Birds and the Bees* will help make all this possible.

2

◆

Laying the Groundwork for Healthy Sexuality

Just how early should parents begin to worry about their child's sexuality? At what age does a child's sexuality begin to develop? These are questions I am often asked by concerned parents.

Your child's sexuality begins to develop from the moment he or she is born. Long before your child begins to have erotic feelings or fantasies, long before he or she begins to masturbate or become attracted to others, he or she is learning about sex and love. He or she is learning about physical pleasure, trust, impulse control, physical and emotional intimacy—all components of sexuality.

While it may be difficult to view your child as a sexual being, one thing is perfectly clear—your child's sexual *potential* is strongly affected by early childhood experiences. Children are indeed sexual—not in the same way as adults, but they have feelings in their genitals, they are developing a sexual identity, sexual attitudes and preferences, and are having sexual experiences.

Our sexual behavior as adults, like most of what we do, springs from the way we feel about ourselves, about others, and about life itself and can be traced to feelings, instincts, attitudes, and personality patterns that first begin to take shape in infancy. From the very beginning, infants begin to develop feelings and attitudes about themselves, their world, and the people close to them that will influence their sexual behavior throughout their lives. Surprisingly, babies do some of their most significant learning about sex and love in the first months of life.

There are many factors influencing your child's sexual development, including whether or not there is adequate bonding between mother and infant; messages you give your child about sex, his or her body, appearance, and gender; the amount and type of affection in the home; and whether or not his or her privacy and personal limits are respected.

EMOTIONAL AND PHYSICAL BONDING

The single most important thing parents can do for their child regarding both emotional and sexual development is to establish a strong emotional bond with their infant. This emotional bond sets the tone for your child's ability to be physically and emotionally intimate later on in life. In fact, physical and emotional bonding are so important that if a child does not receive adequate amounts of it, he or she is likely to be doomed to a life of emptiness and detachment from emotional connectedness.

Children who experience emotional bonding with a parent are far more capable of experiencing emotional intimacy when they become adults than those who did not experience sufficient bonding. In turn, those who are able to experience emotional intimacy are far more likely to develop healthy sexual responses than those who do not.

What exactly is bonding, and how do parents go about establishing an emotional bond with their infant? Bonding is a spontaneous emotional connection that occurs between parent and infant. This physical and emotional connectedness begins with eye contact, caressing, and holding.

For some parents it occurs the moment they first set eyes

on their newborn. For others, it occurs within the first few weeks of their infant's life, during the time when parent and child "become acquainted." Sadly, for other parents, bonding does not occur at all.

Those parents who themselves had parents who were able to bond with them will most likely be able to bond with their infant without any difficulty. In fact, it probably happens automatically without any effort on their part at all. On the other hand, those parents whose own parents did not bond with them may find it extremely difficult to bond with their infant, no matter how hard they try. While they may be happy to have a child, may think the baby is adorable, and may even feel they love the child, something seems to be missing—a kind of deep, heartfelt, emotional connection. They find it difficult to give what they themselves were not given.

What are the roadblocks to healthy emotional bonding between a parent and a child?

Negative reactions to arousal. Some parents, upset by their own or their baby's reaction to stimulation, feel shame, push their baby away, blame their baby for their own responses, or assign attributes to their child such as seductiveness, evil, or incestuous feelings that simply are not there.

It is normal for a mother to become sexually aroused when she is breast-feeding her baby. Those mothers who know and understand this will feel less concerned or embarrassed by the occurrence than those who are caught completely off guard by their response. For example, some mothers who experience this normal arousal feel that they are "sick" and chastise themselves for their reaction. They are so filled with shame that they put walls up between themselves and their baby, never really letting themselves get too close for fear of an "unnatural bond" occurring between them.

Whether you use the breast or bottle-feed, you may notice your boy baby getting an erection when he's feeding. This is an automatic and normal response. There is no need to stimulate or encourage this, but it is very important that you not *discourage* or interfere with it. Your baby girl may also get a clitoral erection, but this is less noticeable. It is usually accompanied by vaginal lubrication, which can be copious, so it's nice to know enough not to be concerned about it.

It is also normal for you to have sexual dreams about your child, even your infant. This is especially prevalent with first boys. Pregnancy itself brings with it powerful emotions, as does the experience of birth, and your glandular system is going through a period of intense readjustment after nine months of profound changes. Also, you are being confronted several times a day with your baby's genital organs and witnessing entirely normal erections. And so your reactions are not surprising and should not disturb you. Eventually your physiological system will readjust and you will come to see your baby for what he is—your son—and your erotic fantasies will stop bothering you.

Unhealthy projections. Projection is the act of attributing to others those feelings and reactions that we ourselves are having but do not want to acknowledge, or in some cases, feelings that we fear we may have or have had in the past.

For example, I was working with a woman named Cindy who had been for quite some time bulimic (she would binge on food and then force herself to throw up). Although her bulimia was now more under control, she still had a fear of becoming fat and still had a very negative body image. Then she suddenly became pregnant. Naturally, we were both concerned about how she was going to react to her weight gain during pregnancy, but surprisingly, she seemed to cope with it very well. She stopped coming to therapy shortly before her delivery date.

One day several months later, Cindy called and asked to see me, but apologized for the fact that she would have to bring her infant daughter because she didn't have a sitter. Even though I suspected the infant would be a terrible distraction, I agreed to see her. As she filled me in on her responses to having a new baby, her infant girl began to cry. Cindy discreetly began to breast-feed her. As her baby suckled, Cindy said to me, "She's such a little pig, she wants to eat all the time." This was a classic case of projection. Cindy was assigning her own issues with food onto her infant daughter. After only a few minutes of suckling, Cindy pulled her infant away from her breast and said, "You've had enough now." The child instantly began to scream, and Cindy said, "She gets so furious with me when I try to limit her intake, but I want to teach her early on not to overeat."

In addition to setting her daughter up for an eating disorder, Cindy was interfering with the bonding process. In order for an infant to bond in a healthy way to a parent, trust needs to be established. Cindy was preventing her baby from trusting that her mother was going to meet her physical and emotional needs.

Discomfort with touch or intimacy. Those parents who did not receive adequate amounts of touching when they were children or who were emotionally and physically smothered will often feel uncomfortable touching their own children and uncomfortable with too much physical or emotional closeness.

For example, some mothers do have a more difficult time than others with breast-feeding because of nipple tenderness, but for others, breast-feeding their infant feels just too intimate, too smothering. They cannot tolerate the level of intimacy or the feeling of having someone need them so much. They may attribute their difficulty to breast tenderness, when in reality it is their fear of intimacy that is causing their discomfort.

HOW YOUR BABY LEARNS HE OR SHE IS LOVED

Some mothers fall in love with their babies the first moment they see them, while others find that their love grows slowly and gradually. But almost all mothers and caretakers know that babies feel loved when they are held snugly and closely, when they are cuddled and fondled and murmured to. The feel of the mother's skin, the protecting curve of her arm, her smile, and even the soothing sound of her voice as she warms his or her bottle or opens her blouse to feed him or her, tell the baby he or she is safe and loved and lovable.

During feeding time, your baby not only receives physical nourishment, which eases hunger pangs, but receives the gift of emotional nourishment as well. Whether you breast-feed or bottle-feed your baby, this experience can be a deeply satisfying one for both you and your baby. It is how you *feel* about what you are doing that is important. What counts most for your baby's well-being is the degree of intimacy and rapport that binds mother and infant closely together during this time.

When your child is provided with enough nurturing and safety, he or she is taught that intimacy and personal involvement are not to be feared and that opening oneself up psychologically to a significant other is nurturing instead of dangerous. On the other hand, a child who is pushed away, neglected, or smothered by his or her parents' love learns that intimate contact is too risky and may grow up preferring alienation or physical sex to the vulnerability of genuine intimacy.

LEARNING TO COMMUNICATE

There is no right way of loving a baby. Each mother and each infant is a unique individual. Since mother and child are separate entities, each must become acquainted with the other's differences. For example, a gentle, quiet mother may be disconcerted to find she has a very active, "difficult" baby whose cries are lusty and loud. Or a lively, vigorous woman may find herself the mother of a slow, quiet infant who seems to take forever with feeding.

You will need to allow you and your baby to tune in to each other gradually. Eventually you will set up your own private communication system in which your baby will tell you what he or she needs, likes, and doesn't like, and you will find out what your baby's signals mean and learn to respond to them in ways satisfying to both of you.

FRUSTRATION AND IMPULSE CONTROL

When you are anxious, your baby may tense up, tighten her or his little limbs and muscles, and begin to kick and howl. Your baby responds to your emotions with her or his whole being. Conversely, when you feel happy and relaxed, your baby is likely to "catch" your contentment. This doesn't mean you have to be relaxed every minute. It is the overall quality of your care that counts in the long run. It is the tender nurturing way in which you minister to his or her distress most of the time that makes your baby feel he or she is loved and wanted.

As an infant gets used to the idea that mother will soon be coming to lessen his or her discomfort, he or she begins to develop a sense of well-being, certainty, and a sense of trust. In time—after the earliest months—a baby becomes confident that mother will appear, and he or she learns to wait a bit for his or her needs to be satisfied. He or she begins to reach out—to explore everything in sight. But it is mother and her warm affection that have set the baby on his or her way to meet the world. In order for a baby to flourish, his or her gratifications and pleasures should outweigh frustrations.

WHERE DOES FATHER COME IN?

With all the emphasis on mother so far, you'd think that fathers have very little importance in a baby's life. But nothing could be further from the truth. Many fathers are almost as active in the physical care of their infants as are mothers. Other fathers, who may not be the most important person in their baby's life from a day-to-day standpoint, nevertheless play a vital role in their infant's development. Their pride in their infant and the extra emotional support they give mother will help her also as she adjusts to her new role in life.

The mutual love between you and your mate (if you have one) can also be an important part of the setting for your baby's healthy emotional and sexual development. The joy and contentment that you experience with one another will radiate toward your baby and warm him or her too.

From a practical viewpoint, babies do not really recognize mother as "Mother" in the earliest months. They respond to whoever represents *mothering* to them. This may mean Dad, Grandma, a babysitter, or any person who is both warm and gentle with them. It is good for babies to get used to one or more other people in their lives from the beginning. Babies feel safe and secure in their father's arms too, and can get that same feeling of well-being and trust when their father gives them the bottle. Warm and special feelings for his or her father as well as for mother will be of great importance in helping shape a baby's future sexual development, attitudes, and behavior.

TOUCH AS SEX EDUCATION

Aside from bonding, there is nothing more important to your child's present or future sexuality than the ability to give and receive touching with trust and spontaneity. The relationship between infant and mother (or other primary caretaker) is the single most important factor contributing to the health, well-being, and eventual sexuality of your child. It is through their mother's (or father's) loving touch that children are given the ability to love themselves and to love others.

By providing your child with a positive experience with touch, physical closeness, and intimacy, you will be laying the groundwork for healthy sexuality in your child.

The intimacy of loving interactions between parent and baby—soothing skin-to-skin experiences, peaceful feeding pleasures, and playful facial games—are actually the child's introduction to bodily pleasure, which is a basic characteristic of sexuality.

Research shows that the amount and the kind of touching we received as infants and young children strongly affects the strength of the adult sex drive and the urge to nurture. For the human being to learn to give love, he or she must first receive it. Each time parents cuddle, hug, rock, or pat a baby or toddler, they give the experience of taking in love. The manner in which the child is touched and treated affects whether he or she finds physical contact pleasurable or not and influences his or her future capacity to enjoy touching and intimacy.

The importance of touching in human life can hardly be overemphasized. Touching is essential for healthy development—in fact the tactile sense is the first to develop. Babies who have not received sufficient tactile stimulation—hugging, cuddling, kissing—do not develop normally and many do not grow at all. In the months following birth, touching can literally mean the difference between life and death; the mortality rate for babies deprived of touching is extremely high.

Most mothers seem to understand this instinctively, providing their infant with a lot of physical contact, but some mothers provide their babies with only the barest of necessities—giving them bottles, changing their diapers, and bathing them—without any real time spent cuddling, admiring, or talking to their infants.

Touching is the simplest, most direct and powerful means of expressing affection, and it is a fundamental part of intimacy, our means of connecting with one another. Perhaps the most important gift parents can give their child is the ability to give and receive touch. Certainly, touching is an essential part of a fulfilled sexual life.

If you can teach your child that to be touched is an enjoyable experience, one that gives pleasure to both parties, one that establishes closeness and trust, then you have laid the groundwork for your child's healthy sexuality.

Parental Messages About Sex

We all received negative messages about sex as we were growing up. But you do not have to pass on to your child the negative messages, fears, and misinformation that were given to you.

Verbal and nonverbal parental messages have a tremendous impact on children and their sexual development. The messages you give your child concerning the importance of touch, her or his genitals, masturbation, the role of sexuality in her or his life, her or his body, intimacy, sex and role identification, sexual orientation, and the stereotypes about males and females all lay the foundation for her or his sexuality. From these early messages, he or she begins to form beliefs about whether sexuality is good or bad, about whether our genitals are "dirty" or not, and ideas about the sexes. These beliefs in turn determine how good or bad your child feels about expressing his or her sexuality and how he or she feels about his or her body, genitals, and gender.

A child's training about sex begins fairly early. The earliest and most deeply influential messages your child will ever receive about sex will be from you, the child's parent.

MESSAGES REGARDING GENITALS

The way you handle your child's early body explorations will have a marked effect on his or her attitude toward his or her body. For example, when a baby boy delights in the discovery of his feet, his mother is usually warmed by his enthusiasm, and yet when the same baby discovers his penis and tries to examine it the same way, mother may grow tense and push his hand away. In this way she is teaching her child that certain parts of the body are taboo.

Every child forms attitudes toward his or her genitals, and these attitudes color his or her view of sex. If a child's parents believe the organs for elimination and reproduction are shameful or nasty, these beliefs will be communicated to their child, and he or she will likely develop similar reactions.

Typically toddlers are taught the correct names for all body parts except the genitals. This inability to apply straightforward names to sexual organs contributes to a sense of mystery about sex—simultaneously bestowing it with importance and shame. My client Melanie told me about how her family handled this issue:

> In our family we had silly names for our genitals. We called them our pee-pees, and the boys' penises were called wienies. This continued up until we were teenagers. Although at school we were learning words like vagina and penis, our parents continued to use these cute names. Mother would always say, 'I have to use the little girl's room,' when she had to go to the bathroom and, 'I have my visitor,' when she started her period. All this tended to give me the message that my genitals and our natural bodily functions are shameful, and I tend to still feel this today.

Parents don't have to say a word in order to communicate their attitude about genitals. It can all happen nonverbally—a mother's facial expression when she changes a diaper, her obvious distaste when her child wants to show her his bowel movement, her anger when her two-year-old daughter wants to examine her vulva. These and other reactions tell children that their genitals are unacceptable, that elimination is dirty. Each time you toilet train, bathe, or dress your child, your attitudes toward his or her body generally and genitals specifically are being communicated to the child.

MESSAGES ABOUT MASTURBATION

It is disheartening to note that even in today's permissive environment, children are still raised to be ashamed of their bodies, their genitals, and their natural body urges such as masturbation. Some genital play is a part of normal development, and the ability to continue to give ourselves sexual pleasure is an important part of developing positive feelings about ourselves sexually. Therefore, if a child's experience with masturbation is positive, it sets the stage for a lifetime of pleasurable masturbation and other sexual experiences.

Since children and adolescents lack knowledge about sex,

their bodies, and their sexual organs, the most basic form of learning about their bodies is to touch and explore them. Those children who feel free to masturbate and explore their bodies and their sensations are better equipped to communicate their needs later on in life to their sexual partners.

If such exploration is handled unwisely by the parent, though, a child will conclude that the genitals and the feelings coming from them are bad and wrong, and this can set the tone for how the child feels about it for the rest of her or his life.

What You Should Know About Masturbation

Beginning in the womb, boys experience an erection and girls experience vaginal lubrication every ninety minutes. This normal sexual phenomenon continues until toilet training. It is quite normal for infants to touch and play with their bodies. It is crucial that you allow your child this natural exploration, which lays the foundation for discovering that the body is good and begins the development of a positive attitude toward sexuality.

There are three stages of normal development during which masturbation occurs almost universally. During infancy, healthy, alert children investigate the genital area with the same curiosity that they experience when they poke at their ears. Since the nerve endings around the genital area are quite sensitive, infants naturally experience a generalized pleasant sensation. This feeling is not the intensely exciting feeling of the mature adult.

Between the ages of three and five, another period of genital play can occur. This is often motivated by an emotional attachment to the opposite-sex parent. Children handle some of their sexual feelings at this stage by self-manipulation. (We will discuss this more later in the book.) Because boys have a noticeable organ for elimination that is pleasurable to touch, they are more apt to play with themselves than girls.

The third period of self-manipulation occurs in adolescence, when the specific activity of the sex glands makes itself felt. Because direct outlets for sexual expression are restricted until adolescents are older, they turn to masturbation to handle the new intensity of their feelings.

Some genital play, then, is a part of normal development. In addition, the ability to continue to give ourselves sexual pleasure is an important part of developing positive feelings about ourselves sexually.

Boys tend to begin masturbating earlier than girls, perhaps because their genitals are so much more accessible. Boys normally begin to masturbate regularly at anywhere from seven to twelve years old. Girls, on the other hand, vary more in terms of when they begin to masturbate. Some girls tend to explore their bodies more than others, and some may discover pleasurable feelings in their genitals when they are horseback-riding, bicycling, running, or playing on monkey bars. Other girls don't explore their genitals or haven't had the experience of accidentally stimulating their clitoris and so do not begin masturbation unless they are taught by other children, introduced to it inappropriately by an adult, or until they enter into sexual relationships with their peers.

How to Handle Your Own Discomfort

Sooner or later, as a part of your child's normal growth to sexual maturity, he or she is going to discover that he or she derives a pleasurable sensation when touching and handling his or her genitals. Because it feels so good, he or she is likely to want to repeat this pleasant experience. And so it should be, except for our society's taboos and restrictions that decree otherwise.

There probably are few words in the English language that cause people more discomfort than the word *masturbation*. Even though we know quite well that masturbating is not wrong, we're likely to feel uneasy, perhaps even distressed, at finding our own child thus occupied.

Those raised in deeply religious households often experience tremendous guilt and shame about masturbation. Touching ourselves and exploring "down there" has been especially discouraged by religious teachings. Masturbation, while practiced by almost everyone, is considered depraved and sinful by many religious organizations.

Obviously, when you do find your child handling his or her genitals, you can't toss aside your own emotions or past upbringing overnight. But you can try to detach yourself somewhat from your feelings and avoid acting hastily—though this may take real doing. When you're able to look at the situation with reasonable objectivity, it will become easier for you to act in the best interest of your child.

What to Do and Say

Most of us know that it is a myth that masturbation causes pimples, impotence, sterility, eye diseases, or any of the long list of ills once attributed to it. But few parents know that although it does not cause insanity or emotional illness, a child may suffer some psychological harm if he or she is made to feel unduly anxious, guilty, or fearful about masturbating.

When young children seem to handle themselves just occasionally, it is not difficult to ignore it. Those children who are happy and active with playmates and with interesting things to do don't take an exaggerated interest in their own bodies. In the normal course of events, it becomes a private matter for them and one needing no further investigating. Sometimes younger children will clutch at their genitals when they are tense or fearful; at other times they may clutch them when they need to urinate. This is not the same as masturbation, and unless it seems chronic, it is wise to ignore it.

It can be embarrassing for parents and for everyone, however, to see a child handling himself or herself openly in the presence of others. Instead of rushing over in panic, take a deep breath, wait a moment, and then simply suggest to your child in a friendly way to wait until he or she is alone to do that and then help him or her find some interesting things to do.

You can say quite calmly (even though you may not feel so calm inside), "I know that feels good, dear, but we don't touch our private parts in front of people. We do that in private." If your child asks, "Why?" you can simply explain that other people don't like to see us do it, that just as we go to the bathroom in private, we touch ourselves in private.

Your child will catch on quickly that touching his or her private parts in public is socially unacceptable. Other children will tease her or him for doing it, and he or she will soon notice that adults and older children don't play with their genitals in public, and this will reinforce your message. Most children seem to develop their own qualms about touching their genitals in front of others without any prompting from parents.

Of course, if your child continues this behavior after age five or so, you may need to do some further investigation. Check to make sure she or he doesn't have a medical or emotional problem of some kind. Ask your child if he or she is aware of touching his or her genitals in public, and if so, ask if the child knows why he or she does so. Ask if her or his genitals feel sore, and check to see if the child has a rash or other skin breakout. If so, she or he may need medical care. A word of caution: Sometimes genital clutching or fondling in public (after age five) can be an indication of childhood sexual abuse.

Even the best-intentioned parent sometimes threatens a masturbating child with a slap or a yank or by punishing her or him, but these measures aren't very successful. They are more likely to lower a child's self-esteem and possibly make her or him feel shameful or unworthy, for a child has no way of knowing that these urges are normal or natural. Instead, your child needs constructive help in curbing his or her actions.

MESSAGES ABOUT SEX PLAY AND SEX TALK

At some time or another, your child's natural curiosity will undoubtedly lead him or her into checking out the anatomy of friends, most particularly those of the opposite sex. This research, often disguised as the well-known game of "doctor," usually takes place behind the closed doors of bedrooms, bathrooms, and closets, indicating that children sense there might be some adult disapproval of their activities.

While many parents are shocked when they discover their child engaged in this kind of mutual inspecting and touching, if you are honest with yourself, you can remember a time when you participated in similar experiments. This is a normal developmental episode for preschool children (ages three to five). The most important thing is for you not to lose your cool. Instead, state your objections very gently, such as, "I know you are having fun, but those things are for when you're all grown up." Explain that his or her genitals are private and that if he or she has any questions, you'd be happy to answer them. Do not send the other child home or make a scene of it.

In fact, children usually want to be stopped because they become uncomfortable and uneasy with the sexual excitement they begin to feel during this kind of play. Once children have embarked on this activity, however, it is hard for them to stop it all by themselves. They actually want you to intervene, and they frequently lead themselves subconsciously into a situation where they're sure to get "caught in the act."

You can put an end to the activity without making your child feel bad. If you scold, punish, or shame your child, it can increase his or her anxiety and actually make the whole idea seem even more enticing. If you simply suggest quietly and firmly that the children should stop this play, your child is likely to feel quite relieved. You can then suggest that they get started on some other activity or you can even help them to find one. In the future you may also want to discourage unsupervised play of twosomes and threesomes behind closed doors.

Later on that day you can point out to your child that, while it is natural for a boy to want to see how girls are made, and for a girl to see how boys are made, there are other ways of finding out than through these games. Encourage your child to talk over with you some of her or his questions about sex differences. You might draw a sketch, or let her or him watch a baby being diapered. In addition, your child may need reassurance that the way he or she is built is right for a boy, or right for a girl.

MESSAGES ABOUT SEX AND ROLE IDENTIFICATION

When a baby is born, our first question often is, "What is it? Is it a boy or a girl?" Research has shown that beginning as early as infancy, girl babies are treated differently than boy babies. Girls are spoken to in a soft, melodic, or high voice, while boys are spoken to in a deeper, rougher voice. Girls are treated as if they are more fragile than boys, while boys are treated in a rougher manner and expected not only to accept the roughness but to like it. These kinds of behaviors are subtle but nevertheless extremely influential.

For many years, it was assumed that gender identity—the sense of oneself as male and masculine or female and feminine—was determined biologically. But now it is believed that while biology is influential, it alone does not dictate gender identity. How parents react to the sex of their infant is also a vital cause of the toddler's early gender sense.

It may be less popular these days for children to be identified in terms of dress—blue for boys and pink for girls—but stereotyping remains a fact of life for many youngsters. We see it in terms of behavior identified as appropriate only for girls or only for boys. Boys and girls still get the impression that it is inappropriate to "act" like a member of the opposite sex.

Many parents worry about sexual confusion and sexual identity, and this is perfectly understandable, especially today with all the discussion about transsexuality and transvestitism. Even liberal parents can become concerned when their little boy appears to enjoy dressing up in feminine clothing. There is somewhat less concern for girls who take on "tomboyish" traits. Most often such behavior is a transitional stage and nothing more. The best thing you can do is see what happens if you don't make an issue of it. If these cross-sexual traits maintain themselves over a long period of time, they may indicate gender confusion. But generally speaking, there is no reason for concern if your child seems to be developing normally in all other areas of his or her life. For example, a child who does well in school, makes friends, and is relatively free of symptoms of emotional maladjustment such as stuttering, failure to thrive, or extreme withdrawal or introversion—and who, at the same time, takes on the behavior, dress, or attitudes of the opposite sex (even in terms of the popular stereotypes), is not a child you need to be concerned about. That child may, in fact, be evidencing a background for creativity and good emotional development, as was true with Marlon:

> From the time I was seven or eight years old, I knew I was different from other kids. While my brothers wanted to play baseball and war, I preferred to spend time with my sisters and their friends, playing house and dressing up. My father really didn't like it, and he gave me a really hard time about it. So when he was around, I'd play with my brothers just to please him. Then, when I was older I really got into art. I could sit for hours drawing and painting and be as happy as could be. But my father told me it was for sissies and tried to get me to stop. He made me feel bad about myself because I wasn't on the baseball teams or the basketball teams the way my brothers were.

Marlon grew up to be an accomplished artist. He is a very well-balanced young man who enjoys women both romantically and as friends.

Most parents encourage their child to accept that they are male or female and learn the differences between male and female behaviors. For instance, when children discover that they cannot be both girl and boy, they are often confused and disappointed. A two-year-old boy may play "mommy," put on her clothing, or declare that he will grow up to be a mother. These behaviors and the feelings underlying them are temporary, however, as the boy's misconceptions are quickly and routinely corrected. Repeated positive interactions with both parents regarding one's particular sex minimizes any unhappiness. It also becomes clear to him that his emerging male gender-role behaviors please both his mother and father, as evidenced by comments like: "That's my boy!" "What a big boy you are!"

In order to accept the label "boy," the child has to accept being different from mother and accept the fact that his future is tied to maleness. A mother can promote male gender-role behavior in her son by subtlely encouraging him to be different from her. Fathers usually play a subtle, supportive role in this process if they are loving models for sons to identify with and if they take an active role in their upbringing. However, if the mother has a need to prolong the infantile closeness with her son, she may cause the toddler to be afraid of trying new things, taking part in rough-and-tumble play, and being a boy.

Jason's mother, Emily, inadvertently caused him to be effeminate because of her deep hostility toward males. Emily grew up hearing her mother constantly complain about "good-for-nothing men." Jason's parents fought frequently over the fact that his father spent too much time out drinking with the "boys." All during Jason's childhood, his mother gave him the message that to be male was to be selfish and unreliable, traits that Jason remembers feeling strongly that he did not want to have. This and his father's lack of involvement with him caused Jason to reject any innate "male" behaviors that he might naturally exhibit and to take on more effeminate mannerisms in order to please his mother.

Traumatic events and troubled families can discourage a child from accepting the biologically appropriate label. A father's drunken rages may frighten a young boy about growing up to be a man. A mother's harshness and disinterest may also leave her son frightened about maleness and uncertain as to how to elicit affection.

Many children are given the parental message that they are the wrong sex. Because they are helpless to alter it, their feeling that their particular sex is second-best tears at children's self-respect in a devastating way, making them feel unacceptable at a very basic level. Part of any child's high self-esteem is feeling "I'm glad I'm a girl," or "I'm glad I'm a boy." If his or her parents are not happy with a child's sex, the child certainly cannot be. A small percentage of children who develop conspicuous disturbances in gender identity were once treated by their families as though they were members of the opposite sex, as was the case with Sloan.

Sloan's parents had already had three female children by the time she was born. Each time her mother became pregnant, her father was certain that this time he was going to get the boy he so longed for, and each time he was terribly disappointed. When Sloan was born, it seemed that her father just couldn't cope with one more disappointment, and so, beginning with her name, he began treating her like a boy. Sloan's mother just didn't have the heart to tell her husband he was out of line.

By the time she was three, Sloan had become her father's sidekick. He took her with him fishing, camping, and hiking. He taught her how to play softball and fought to have her included in boys' Little League where he was the coach. Sloan watched her dad while he worked on the family car, and by the time she was a teenager, thanks to his teaching, she was a first-rate mechanic.

When other girls began to take an interest in dressing up for boys, Sloan thought they were all crazy. She had better things to do, like working on projects with her father in the garage, or taking off on hiking trips. All during high school she was a star athlete on the track team. She hated the home economics classes she was required to take and fought successfully to take shop instead. She was popular with both the boys and the girls, but no one ever asked her out on a date, and she was secretly glad no one did.

In college, however, things started to get more confusing for Sloan. Away from her parents and the group of friends who had become accustomed to her differentness, she became more uncomfortable with the fact that she was expected to date men but really didn't want to. And while her tomboy ways had been tolerated and even considered "cute" among her family and friends, in college she began to be ridiculed. Many of her classmates thought she was a lesbian, and one lesbian friend made a sexual pass at her.

This last event is what brought Sloan into therapy. She was extremely upset by her friend's sexual approach and what it meant in terms of her sexual orientation. Before the first session was over, however, Sloan confessed to me that in fact she didn't think she was a lesbian, but that she felt like a male. I explained to Sloan that she was what professionals call "male identified," meaning that in all respects, she identified with men far more than with women. As it turned out, Sloan was so confused about her gender identity that she had no sexual desire for men or women, and this bothered her immensely because she wanted to have a family later on in life.

The formation of core gender identity does not suddenly happen; it gradually emerges from a seeming gender neutrality in early life. While a fifteen-month-old boy has more in common with all toddlers than with boys in particular, he has already begun learning about and identifying with males. His sense of himself as a boy will progressively appear during the next year or so. The sex of the child begins as a powerful factor in the parents' minds, but by the first birthday it is becoming a powerful factor in the child's mind. Another key factor, therefore, of core gender identity is the quality of the child's relationships early in life.

Although there has been a trend in the last ten years or so toward "unisex" identification of children and a deemphasis on labeling toys and activities as "male" or "female," recent research shows that most girls, if given the choice between playing with dolls or with trucks, will choose to play with dolls. And most boys, given the same choice, will choose to play with trucks. The important thing is not to be too rigid in either direction, neither insisting on your child playing and acting in sex-appropriate ways, nor insisting on his or her breaking out of stereotypical roles. Allow your child to develop naturally, to take part in whatever games or activities he or she is interested in, regardless of his or her "sex." Do not try to impose your will on your child.

MESSAGES ABOUT SEXUAL ORIENTATION

The second landmark of sexual identity development after gender identification is the establishment of sexual orientation. Many parents are concerned about making sure their child does not become homosexual. Some fathers are so concerned that they are reluctant to be affectionate with their sons after age five or six for fear that the child will become homosexual. This is unjustified and very distressing to the child. Other parents overreact to their children's play when it does not conform to long-standing stereotypes—for example, when boys play dress-up in women's clothing or play with dolls, or when girls play tough and like sports—as discussed earlier.

Most professionals agree that there's nothing parents can do to prevent their children from becoming homosexual. No specific attitudes or behaviors have been found to discourage the development of a homosexual orientation. Similarly, there is no convincing evidence that parents can cause homosexuality in their children.

On the other hand, our culture continually steers children toward heterosexuality through messages from the family, the schools, the media, and peer relationships. Children's erotic preoccupations are directed toward heterosexuality by their need to obtain and retain the approval of others. And children learn to hide any homoerotic impulses or feelings when they see the negative, anxious responses they produce in parents, teachers, and friends.

Therefore, the chances are far more likely that your child will become heterosexual than homosexual. On the other hand, if it turns out that your child is homosexual, you don't want to discourage him or her from coming forward and telling you or from feeling good about himself or herself as a result of your negative attitudes about homosexuality. Therefore, try to convey an attitude of acceptance for people who have different sexual orientations. Otherwise, your child may grow up to feel like Adam did:

> It's taken me years to finally learn to accept my homosexuality, in spite of the fact that my father does not. He made it perfectly clear from the time I was around nine years old that he could never accept me if I was a homosexual. But with the help of a gay support group and lots of loving friends, I have finally learned not just to accept my gayness but to be genuinely proud of it. I've stopped acting straight just to pacify my father, and that feels especially good.

ATTITUDES ABOUT THE SEXES

Another message your child receives, from both the family and from society in general, is how males and females are to be perceived. Your attitudes about the sexes directly affect your child's feelings about herself or himself and can severely interfere with her or his relationships with the opposite sex. Spend some time thinking about your own mother's attitude about men and your father's attitude about women. Also think about the attitudes about the sexes that permeated your environment.

A good way of discovering what your attitude is about the opposite sex is to look at the words you use to identify them. If you grew up hearing your parents or your peers talk about the opposite sex in derogatory terms, it is likely that you adopted these same terms and, consequently, the same attitudes. Many women, themselves raised among men who used these derogatory words to describe females, seem to take these terms for granted. This was the case with Bonnie:

> My father used very derogatory words when referring to sex and female genitalia in particular. I was keenly aware from the time I was very small that he did not respect women— that he only saw them as objects to be used. Naturally this made me feel ashamed to be a female, ashamed of my body, especially my genitals.

Melinda's mother also passed on her negative attitudes about men to her daughter, which in turn ended up influencing Melinda's attitudes about men and sex:

My mother warned me from the time I was very young that all men wanted was sex. I never thought of sex as pleasurable for the woman—it was just a thing you put up with if you wanted to have a man, or something you used to bargain with to get things you wanted.

Consequently, because Melinda went into each sexual experience with no expectations of pleasure, but with the attitude of "When is this going to be over?" she had no chance to experience enjoyable sex. This further reinforced her mother's message. By the time Melinda came into therapy, she had become so cut off from her body that she suffered pain whenever she had intercourse.

Sometimes both parents, and in fact the entire family, will teach children to have a particular attitude about the sexes. This was the case in Angela's family:

My entire family preferred males. When a male was born it was time for celebration; when a female was born condolences were in order. I grew up envying males and feeling less than any male I had contact with.

We are also trained by family and society about how our own sex is expected to act and how our sex is perceived by others. Females are often trained to be seductive and sexy and to derive their good feelings from winning male approval and turning men on, while at the same time remaining virginal and innocent.

Males, on the other hand, are supposed to be aggressive and experienced. While girls are still guaranteed a bad reputation for being sexually curious or sexually active, boys are guaranteed admiration for the exact same behavior. This puts some boys in a precarious position of having to find a girl to have sex with them even if they aren't ready for the experience.

Contraceptive pills and the sexual revolution have caused

some parents to become more permissive with their female children, but even today our culture is still steeped in the belief that young men need to sow their wild oats while girls should beware of becoming "used property." Many a father is secretly proud of his son's sexual escapades, believing that they underscore his son's virility. Promiscuity in boys is more likely to be sanctioned by society; "Boys will be boys!" we say. But male promiscuity has nothing to do with masculinity. It has far more to do with low self-esteem, insecurity about masculinity, and disrespect for females, and it may be a symptom of child sexual abuse.

RELIGIOUS MESSAGES ABOUT SEX

Although we live in the twentieth century, the archaic belief that sex is evil and dirty still lurks in our minds. We may not consciously admit to this outmoded view, but we certainly act as if we believe it.

In the fifteenth and sixteenth centuries in Europe, earthly pleasure was regarded as sinful. Sex was seen as necessary for the continuation of the race, but enjoyment of it was publicly viewed as the work of the devil. Sex symbolized mankind's fall. Even between a married couple, sex was meant for procreation only. Sex brought out the beast in man; and if a woman enjoyed sex, it meant she was immoral and depraved.

Western religion today, based on Judeo-Christian ideas of morality, still teaches us that sex is primarily intended for procreation. The traditional Christian view of the body is that it is the source of all temptation and sin. Rather than being considered a sacred vessel of the divine, the body is seen as a vehicle for the profane, with a relentless potential for sin.

Tammy grew up in a very religious household. Most of the family's activities were centered around going to church. Very early on she learned that sex was the work of the devil. The women in her congregation were not allowed to wear makeup, and they were required to wear their dresses below their knees and never to wear short sleeves. Dancing was not permitted because it was seen as the devil's way of tempting them, and they were also forbidden to go to the movies or to listen to rock-and-roll music for the same reason.

It is no surprise that when Tammy got married she was unable to have intercourse with her husband. Like so many other women raised in religions where sex is seen as evil, Tammy could not suddenly switch from being a woman who felt that any sexual reaction on her part was sinful, to allowing herself to open up sexually with her husband.

Whatever your religious beliefs, be aware that religious messages can affect how a child perceives his or her body and his or her natural sexual curiosity and feelings.

MESSAGES FROM DIVORCE

Today's typical family is seldom the stereotypical mother, father, brother, and sister. Divorce is so common that two-household families are almost becoming the norm. Parents need to be careful not to blame their ex-spouse, complain about him or her in front of their children, or tell secrets about him or her to their children. This kind of behavior models to children that there is always a "good guy" and a "bad guy" in relationships and that people can't be trusted with our vulnerability and our secrets.

THE BENEFITS OF EARLY SEX EDUCATION

In addition to all the verbal and nonverbal parental messages about sex already discussed, your children will learn your attitudes about sex based on when and how you begin to discuss sex with them. If you avoid sexual discussions, they will interpret this to mean that you are ashamed of sex, that sex is not a subject to be discussed openly, but something to be hidden. If, on the other hand, you begin to discuss sex with your children very early on in an open and relaxed way, you will be passing on the attitude that sex is natural, wholesome, and healthy. Ensuring that children grow up to be adults capable of making healthy decisions about their sexuality calls for a parent-child dialogue that should begin much earlier than most parents would expect. Sexual learning is a lifelong process; sexual teaching begins for parents at the birth of their first child and continues to unfold as the child's needs grow and change.

Unfortunately, most parents do not discuss sex with their children in an open, calm way. Instead, parents communicate their fears, discomfort, and embarrassment about sexuality to their children.

In the typical family, parents teach only the mechanics of sex and spend very little time discussing either the responsibilities that go along with sex or the issues of intimacy and caring. Most parents give their children incomplete and confusing information about their sexual development, inadequate sex education, and little or no information about what they can expect during sexual experiences. And many parents feel a great deal of shame and embarrassment about sex, and this is communicated to their children, who in turn internalize their feelings of shame. If parents seem ashamed, embarrassed, or confused about discussing sex, a child's chances of developing a healthy sexual identity are probably limited. Most people in our society have no consistent model for or firsthand experience of healthy sexuality.

On the other hand, some parents react against their own puritanical upbringing by providing their children with too much information about sex and too much permission to explore their sexuality. Some mothers who consider themselves enlightened provide their daughters with the pill and then retreat into the background, and some parents go so far in the opposite direction from how they were raised that they end up encouraging their children to be promiscuous.

PARENTAL ISSUES:
TOUCH AND SEXUAL MESSAGES

It is vitally important to discover the issues you may have that interfere with your giving your children adequate touching and positive messages regarding sex and their bodies. It is important to discover just which negative messages you received when you were growing up, which messages you still believe, and which ones you are likely to pass on to your children.

The following questions and exercises will enable you to have a better understanding about your sexual attitudes and help you to focus on changing those attitudes and beliefs that may interfere with your child's healthy sexual development.

TOUCH

While it is difficult to determine whether or not you received adequate touching and nurturing as an infant and small child, most of us have an internal sense of how much touching we received. In addition, you can begin to put the pieces of the puzzle together by remembering and noticing the following:

+ How much do you remember being touched and held by your parents throughout your childhood?
+ Are your parents affectionate with you now?
+ How free do you feel to be affectionate with those you are close to?
+ Were you able to bond with your own children when they were infants?
+ Were you or are you able to be affectionate with your own children?

SEXUAL MESSAGES

Negative messages about sex, genitals, masturbation, gender identity, and sexual orientation can affect our sexuality immensely because we end up believing things that are not only untrue, but that hamper our sexual spontaneity, make us feel bad about our normal sexual urges, and make us feel shame about our bodies.

Your sexuality, which includes your most basic ideas of what sex is, what it means, and how and when it is appropriate, was formed early in your life, most notably by your family experiences where you began to absorb the messages about sex that would stay with you all of your life. It is vital, therefore, that you work on remembering just what those messages were, how they affected you, and most importantly, which of them you still believe and which ones you need to discard in order to make room for healthier, more sexually liberating ones. Remembering and gathering information about the messages you received from your family, from religion, and from society in general regarding sex will help you to understand more about your own sexual attitudes and where they come from.

◆

EXERCISE

Parental Messages

◆ List all the messages, both verbal and nonverbal, that you remember receiving from your parents regarding sex. Try to recall not only verbal messages, but also behaviors, attitudes, and specific incidents that also reflected your parents' attitudes regarding sex.

◆ If you are having some difficulty, the following questions may help spark your memory:

1. How did your parents express their affection toward one another?
2. Were your parents ever overtly sexual with one another in front of you?
3. Did your father ever make jokes about how difficult it was to get your mother to have sex, or complain about how he "never got enough"?
4. Did your mother act as if sex was a burden she had to endure or complain about how your father could never get enough?
5. How did your parents handle sex education?
6. How did your parents respond to you as you developed

sexually? (Was it considered a natural right of passage or a negative experience?)
7. Did your parents caution you against premarital sex?
8. Was there a double standard for the boys and the girls in the family (okay for boys to have premarital sex, not okay for girls)?
9. What was your parents' attitude about unmarried couples living together?

What If You Don't Remember Any Messages About Sex?

Talking to your own parents about the messages they gave you regarding sex may prove to be helpful. Even though you and they may feel embarrassed talking to one another about sex, now that you are an adult, your parents may find it easier to talk about their uneasiness and embarrassment about sex than when you were a child. They may have become more knowledgeable, enlightened, and flexible regarding sex and may welcome the chance to apologize to you about the negative or inaccurate messages they passed on to you. In addition, they may be able to share with you information about the messages they themselves received from their parents. This information will not only put things in perspective, but can provide you valuable information regarding some of the beliefs you have about sex that you don't actually remember hearing from your parents directly but have acted on nevertheless.

Sexual Messages Checklist

Which of the following messages about sex did you receive either from your parents, other family members, society in general, or from your church?

1. Touching the genitals is bad.
2. Sexual pleasure is bad.
3. Sexuality is animalistic.

4. The genitals are dirty and are organs to be ashamed of.
5. Sex is something to be endured.
6. Sex is something "nice" people don't enjoy.
7. Don't look, dress, act, or feel sexy.
8. Sexual secretions are dirty.
9. Using sex to hurt others is okay.
10. Withholding sex is a good way to get even.
11. Something is wrong with you if you don't experience an orgasm with every sexual act.
12. You should not enjoy sex—it is for procreation only.
13. You should not enjoy foreplay.
14. Masturbation is evil.
15. Masturbating your partner is evil.
16. Only men should be sexually aggressive.
17. It is only important for a man to have an orgasm, not a woman.

Which of these messages do you still believe (in spite of all you've heard to the contrary) and which ones do you think still influence your sexual attitudes and behavior in negative ways? Work on turning these negative messages into more healthy ones. For example: "The genitals are dirty and are organs to be ashamed of" can be changed into "The genitals are a natural part of the body that serve important functions and provide great physical pleasure." Practice saying these more positive messages to yourself as a first step toward replacing the negative ones in your mind.

If you lay the proper foundation for your child's sexuality by emotionally and physically bonding, by providing loving touch and acceptance, by working on not passing on negative messages about sex, and by providing positive early sex education, your child will begin his or her sex life with positive, healthy attitudes concerning sexuality, and this will in turn help him or her to establish intimate, caring relationships later on.

3

Sex and the Family

Next to parental bonding and parental messages, the most significant influence on a child's sexuality is the relationships within the family. It is within the context of the family that a child learns her or his first lessons about how to treat the opposite sex, how to communicate needs to her or his partner, how to set limits, and the importance of respecting personal privacy.

MODELING ATTITUDES AND
COMMUNICATION SKILLS

Parents' attitudes toward each other will most certainly affect their child's attitude about the opposite sex. If you and your mate treat each other with respect and consideration, you are modeling how your child should treat his or her future partner. On the other hand, if you treat your spouse with disrespect, you are not only modeling this behavior in the family but are teaching your child to disrespect males or females in general.

If there is harmony in the family, if each person is treated with respect and honesty, then children will learn very important lessons concerning how they should treat those they care about, how they should expect others to treat them, and how an intimate relationship should function. On the other hand, if there is a great deal of chaos, fighting, or other disruptions within the family, children will get their first negative lessons on how to behave toward their mate and how they can expect to be treated by their mate.

What does this have to do with your child's sexuality? Everything. An important component of a healthy sexual relationship is a balance of power. In order for a couple to have a healthy sexual relationship, they must be equals in each other's eyes. If your female child learns from you that women are less than men, she will feel inadequate compared to men, will allow men to control her, and will feel desperate to get their attention. If she learns by your example that she can expect to be treated poorly by her mate, she will attract men who use her, are unfaithful to her, or neglect her needs. And if she learns from you that it is okay to put up with disrespectful or even abusive behavior from your mate, then she will grow up to follow your example. If, on the other hand, she is raised to believe that men and women are equal, that both should treat each other with respect, and that it is unacceptable to allow your mate to treat you abusively (whether verbally, emotionally, physically, or sexually), then she will grow up to expect this kind of positive treatment from her mate.

Another important lesson your child will learn from your interactions with your mate, as well as from the general interactions in the family, are communication skills. Experts in sexuality have found that one of the main components of a successful sexual relationship is good communication. Those couples who know how to ask for what they want, who regularly take time out to discuss their relationship, and who have learned good methods of conflict resolution, tend to have a better sex life. From watching you and your spouse interact, your child will learn what is acceptable and unacceptable in terms of communicating with girlfriends or boyfriends and future mates. The way you and your mate speak to one another, the way you communicate your needs, the way you resolve conflicts, will all be noted and imprinted in your child's mind.

MODELING A RESPECT FOR PERSONAL PRIVACY

Parents can also give negative messages about sex and intimacy by not respecting their children's personal boundaries. Our boundaries are those physical and emotional barriers that separate us from others and from the world. We need firm boundaries to define us ("This is where you end and I begin") and to prevent us from merging with others.

In unhealthy families, physical boundaries are either overly rigid or enmeshed. Rigid boundaries are like walls between parents and children, giving children the message that touching is not permissible within the family. When children receive these kinds of messages from their parents' behavior ("No one ever touched in my family," "When my parents did hug or kiss us it felt like a duty"), they will undoubtedly grow up to have difficulties learning how to be intimate.

Enmeshed boundaries, on the other hand, give children the message that they do not have a right to their own privacy and separateness or a right to have control over their own bodies. Boundary violations by parents include: exposing children to their parents' sexual behavior; denying privacy to an older child by walking in on her or him in the bathroom or bedroom without knocking; making inappropriate remarks to their children about their bodies and their sexual development; asking teenagers and even young adults about their sexual experiences; talking inappropriately about sex in front of their children.

Children who are raised in homes where there are frequent boundary violations like those listed above are more likely to intrude upon the privacy and personal space of others and to allow others to intrude upon their privacy and personal space.

For example, boys who are allowed to walk in on their mothers or sisters in the bathroom or to go through their mother's or sister's private things are not as likely to respect the privacy of the girls they have contact with. Conversely, girls who are walked in on by their fathers or brothers are more likely to allow boys to touch them even when they don't want to be touched.

Children need to learn that they must respect the privacy and personal space of others. They learn this by their parents' example and by their parents' strong admonitions against boundary violations.

Parents with a blurred, unclear sense of their own and others' boundaries behave in overly intrusive ways that serve to engender an unhealthy form of closeness and intensity of feeling. Children raised in such families don't know how to define their limits and are unable to protect their rights. They lack a healthy sense of separateness and individuality that might enable them to know and to say what feels okay and what doesn't. Such children grow into adults who unconsciously violate others' boundaries and allow others to violate theirs.

In healthy families, sex education is provided, but sex is not talked about in a derogatory or teasing way. There is open affection between the mother and father, but no explicit sexuality is exhibited in front of the children. Individual privacy is respected—especially the child's right to privacy concerning his or her own body and sexual experiences. All family members knock before entering bathrooms and bedrooms.

FAMILY NUDITY

The issue of family nudity is a touchy one. Some experts believe that it is important to establish an appreciation of the nude body as a natural and beautiful object early in childhood. Many argue that excessive modesty inhibits sexuality. Some people have blamed their sexual problems on the fact that there was no open nudity in their childhood home, as Teresa did:

I think that because I was never exposed to nudity in my family, I found it difficult to undress in front of my husband when I first got married. When I was a kid, I never saw either one of my parents naked. I bathed myself from the time I was six years old. Today I still prefer to make love in the dark, and I still don't like anyone seeing me naked, not even my husband.

Many people insist that these kinds of inhibitions concerning nudity are due to the fact that most people are raised without nudity in any form. They argue that in some families nudity is viewed as extremely unnatural, instead of a natural part of living. These people advocate such things as bathing with your child, not covering up just because your child walks into a room and finds you nude, and some even advocate attending family-oriented nudist camps.

For a time, parents were advised by experts that they should be more "natural" about their own bodies in the presence of their children. This was in reaction to years of Victorian prudery when there was a great deal of secrecy about the human body that was indeed unhealthy. Many parents took this to mean that at home they should feel free to go parading about in the nude. This, they thought, would help their children grow up "free and unrepressed."

But instead of this new "openness" helping young children, it tended to arouse more curiosity and some anxiety. This is understandable, since there is a vast difference in the size and appearance of children's genitals compared with those of their parents. The obvious disparities can confuse and even frighten some children. Besides, even a very young boy may show signs of sexual excitement on seeing his mother in the nude. A little girl, too, can be sexually stimulated by the sight of her naked father. There have been some instances of children who wanted to touch and handle what they saw. All of this seems especially to affect the child of three to five, who is still struggling with fantasies of love and possession of the opposite-sex parent and rivalry with the same-sex parent.

Because of the above reactions, parents need to question whether they need to go to the extreme of walking around naked in front of their child in order to instill in their child the idea that the nude body is natural and beautiful. For example, bathing a young child (under five) offers an excellent avenue for communicating the idea that nudity is acceptable and fun. The warmth of the water is very sensual, as is the feel of your hands and the soap. You can even talk to your child about what a fine body he or she has while you wash him or her.

It is also important that we do not equate shame with modesty. You can teach your child modesty without instilling shame about his or her body. A two-year-old who wants to go outside and play with nothing on should not be chastised and made to feel dirty, but should be brought into the house and told that he or she must have clothes on to go outside.

It is natural for children to become modest at around the age of six or seven. Regardless of their environment (whether their parents are modest or believe in open nudity), they begin to insist on taking their own baths and having privacy when they dress.

Children who do not develop a natural sense of modesty by about seven can be told that while there is nothing wrong with the naked body, we cover it when we are in front of other people. And a teenager who wants to walk around the house in his or her underwear can be told that he or she is too old to be doing so—without making him or her feel ashamed of his or her body.

We do not live in a primitive society where open nudity is acceptable. To teach a child otherwise is to confuse him or her and even set an example of rebellion and going against society's rules. If that is your intention, then fine, but if you want your child to stay within the rules of society, especially where sexuality is concerned, then it is important to teach the prevailing rules.

There are, in fact, many other reasons besides modesty for

clothing the body—protection from the elements (heat, cold, rain, and now, ultraviolet rays), hygiene, and to discourage sexual abuse.

Another argument that is sometimes used for family nudity is that if the only nudity children are exposed to while growing up is that in popular magazines, videos, or the movies, the child will develop expectations and values that are totally unreasonable. Since bodies come in various sizes, shapes, and proportions, airbrushed photos and the perfect bodies of models and actors convey the message that nudity is all right only if the nude person is young and perfect.

Unfortunately, children are going to be exposed to that message no matter how much nudity there is at home. It is naive to ignore the role of the media in shaping our children's values and body images. (This role will be discussed in detail in Chapter Four, "Raising a Child with a Healthy Body Image").

There is no reason to feel that the occasional glimpse of a naked parent is going to be traumatic for a child. Parents can use the experience to teach their child about the importance of respecting each other's privacy without making the child feel ashamed or "bad." For example, let's suppose your five-year-old son rushes into the bathroom while you are taking a bath to tell you something important and finds you naked. But in the middle of his story he gets distracted by your naked body. All you need to do is calmly say something like, "It's important to knock on doors to bathrooms and bedrooms before entering. People like to be alone and private at times. I like privacy when I take a bath." It is your general attitude toward nudity, toward sex, and toward your children that are the important factors, and the number of minutes and the number of inches of body exposure are only secondary.

BEDROOM PRIVACY VERSUS "THE FAMILY BED"

Many child psychiatrists and guidance counselors suggest, whenever possible, that parents plan things so that a young child or even a baby won't be sharing their bedroom at night. They believe that when a baby and his or her parents become used to sleeping in the same room, the arrangement is sometimes continued long after it should have been stopped. It is not good for the child, or for his parents.

As hard as it may be for you to believe, when a child sleeping in the same room hears his or her parents having sex, it can leave a vague but disturbing and indelible impression on even a young child. Children are not always as sound asleep as you may think. In the dark, or half dark, they may be confused and stimulated by what they hear or see—or imagine they hear or see. The sounds and movements of their parents' lovemaking may appear to be those of anger or attack instead of love and passion. Even though they may sense that their mother and father share some special kind of physical intimacy, they are not yet prepared to deal with the overwhelming feelings— sexual excitement, as well as jealousy and guilt—that can seize them now.

Generally speaking, most experts believe it is not a good policy to allow children to sleep with parents. There are a few professionals who advocate the "family bed" concept, in which parents are encouraged to have their children sleep with them, even into adulthood. The rationale behind this is that it helps children to bond with parents and to feel more secure and loved. But this behavior is perceived as radical and unnecessary by most experts. There are many other ways to bond and comfort your child, as discussed earlier. And any positive effects are outweighed by the negative effects of children becoming overly dependent and attached to parents and by the risk of childhood sexual abuse. Most experts agree that children need to have their own beds in order to encourage autonomy and that they need to recognize their parents' "adult" relationship. In addition, the "family bed" can wreak havoc with the marital bed. Parents need to maintain their privacy in order to maintain a healthy emotional and sexual relationship.

If your child has traumatic dreams or nightmares and wants the comfort of sleeping with you, it might be a good idea to say, "I'll stay with you for a while until you fall asleep." Or invite the child to come to your bed for a while until comforted, then carry the youngster back to bed.

There is certainly nothing wrong with allowing your child to jump into bed with you in the morning. Sharing this physical affection and warmth provides him or her with a sound basis for the capacity to love and eventually to be a loving parent. You may recall fondly the fun you had wrestling with your parents in bed. Some parents worry about sexual stimulation, but most are quite comfortable with the idea. If you find yourself becoming stimulated by this contact and are able to acknowledge the sensual delight of loving your child so closely without making it an overtly sexual experience, then things are under control. It should become a playful "roughhouse" experience or one of comforting, rather than one that is specifically erotic. But if you or your partner becomes sexually stimulated and then focuses that feeling onto the child, even in fantasy, it will be important that you stop allowing the visits to your bed.

If you are a single parent who has always allowed your child to jump into bed with you, you will need to discontinue this practice when you become involved in a new sexual relationship. Research shows us that children who have a stepfather are twice as likely to be sexually abused than those who do not. In my opinion it is far more important to protect your child from sexual molestation than to allow any of the positive experiences of roughhousing.

In addition, it is difficult enough for a child to adjust to his or her parent's new partner without adding sexuality to the mix. For example, right after her ex-husband left their home two years ago, my client Heather's eight-year-old son, Billy, began coming into her bed in the morning. She felt he needed extra reassurance, and so she allowed him to cuddle up to her. Soon, he was asking if he could sleep with her at night, and once again she complied.

Recently Heather became involved with a new man. When her boyfriend started spending the night, her son continued to come into the bed both in the morning and sometimes at night before bed. Not surprisingly, Billy and Heather's new boyfriend did not get along well. They had frequent fights, and Billy would sometimes go into rages when asked to do something by the new boyfriend. Heather's boyfriend complained that Billy should not be allowed in the bed, either in the morning or at night.

I advised Heather that it was not a good idea for her son to be in the bed with her for several reasons. First of all, at eight he was too old to be sleeping with his mother. At that age boys often feel erotic feelings toward their mothers, and it can be confusing to have such intimate contact with her. In addition, I felt that Billy saw her new boyfriend as a rival (understandably so) and that having him come into bed with them just exacerbated this rivalry.

By setting clear boundaries regarding nudity and privacy, you as a parent will be taking a significant step toward avoiding a more serious problem, that of emotional incest.

EMOTIONAL INCEST

Emotional or covert incest can be defined as a parent becoming overly involved and overly invested in his or her child's life. This can occur when a child becomes the sole or main focus of a parent's affection, love, and preoccupation. It may take the form of being overly possessive and not wanting your child to have friends or to begin dating. It may take the form of making the child into a sort of "surrogate mate" by treating the child as a primary confidant, friend, and equal partner. Or, it may take the form of seductiveness and intrusion.

When the relationship with the child exists to meet the needs of the parent rather than those of the child, the boundary between caring and incestuous love is crossed. The result is that the child ends up feeling used and trapped. She or he is never able to feel okay about her or his own needs, and attempts at play, autonomy, and friendship outside the home cause the child to feel guilt-ridden and lonely. Over time, the child becomes preoccupied with the parent's needs and feels protective and overly concerned about the parent. Thus, a psychological "marriage" between parent and child results. The child becomes the parent's surrogate spouse.

As a therapist I have heard many clients, both children and adults, make the following comments: "It feels funny to me when my dad worries so much about how I dress and gets jealous when I go out on dates," or "I wish my mother would stop telling me about her problems with my father, it's none of my business," or "I hate it when my dad keeps telling me how much he loves his 'little princess.' " Although the complaints are different, the message is the same: a deep sense of violation by the parent.

The following are examples of inappropriate relationships between a parent and a child:

- ✦ A father frequently complains to his daughter about the difficulties in the marriage. He expresses feelings of loneliness, bitterness, and dissatisfaction with his marriage and his sex life. His child becomes his confidante, and she begins to feel responsible for "cheering up" her father.
- ✦ When boys begin to notice an adolescent girl, her father acts more like a jealous boyfriend than a father. He refuses to let her date until she is eighteen, and then is critical of each boy she goes out with.
- ✦ Many parents walk a fine line between emotional and sexual incest. Even though they do not touch their child inappropriately, they display an unhealthy interest in their child's body either by openly staring at him or her, by taking seductive pictures of the child, by making inappropriate sexual remarks, or by not allowing their child privacy in the bedroom or bathroom.

Even though these violations are usually done in the name of "caring" and "love," there is nothing caring about a close parent-child relationship when it services the needs and feelings of the parent rather than the child. Children should not have to listen to their parents' problems, comfort them when they are lonely, act as a marriage counselor for their parents, or act as their parents' confidant.

Although a child may love being treated as "special" and "privileged" by a parent, being given a special position in the family and idealized by a parent, this same child is cheated out of childhood by serving as a parent's surrogate partner.

The element of seduction inherent in these psychological marriages is subtle and insidious, as is its effect on the child's capacity for a fulfilling sexual and intimate life. Since the parent-child relationship is used to meet the needs of the parent, the child feels ashamed of his or her own legitimate needs. As unhealthy as it is, the child has no choice but to participate actively in meeting the parent's needs while ignoring his or her own. The child already feels emotionally abandoned, and expressing his or her own needs raises the fear of more abandonment. Separation never occurs, and feelings of being trapped in a psychological marriage deepen. This interferes with the child's capacity for healthy intimacy and sexuality.

And last but not least, once the boundary between parent and child is crossed in a covertly incestuous relationship, potential for further victimization in the household exists. For example, if the oldest boy is in a psychological marriage with his mother, he may act out his anger and sexualized energy with a younger sister in an overtly sexual way. (We will discuss the issue of sibling incest later in this chapter.) What started out as a spillover of unmet intimate and sexual needs from the inappropriate relationship with his mother works its way into overt incest between siblings. This example clearly demonstrates how one person's behavior in a family affects the family system as a whole.

Emotional incest occurs most often in two circumstances: in troubled marriages and in single-parent households, or households where one parent is frequently away from home.

Often in troubled marriages, as the deterioration in the marriage progresses, one parent (usually the one of the opposite sex) becomes increasingly dependent on the child, and the relationship is increasingly characterized by desperation, jealousy, and a disregard for personal boundaries. The child becomes the object to be manipulated and used so the parent can avoid the pain and reality of a troubled marriage.

A healthy emotional and sexual bond between parents creates an unspoken, unseen boundary that channels sexual feelings and energies. When a child grows up in a family in which the marriage is chronically disturbed, sexual feelings and energy are never put in perspective, and a psychological marriage with the child may be formed.

To the child, the parent's love feels more confining than freeing, more demanding than giving, and more intrusive than nurturing. The relationship becomes sexually energized and violating, even without the presence of sexual innuendos, sexual touch, or conscious sexual feelings on the part of the parent. The chronic lack of attachment in the marriage is enough to create an atmosphere of sexualized energy that spills over to the child.

In the second situation, that of single-parent households, the parent looks to the child to escape feelings of fear and loneliness of being without a mate. In order to avoid this, single parents need to guard against becoming overly dependent and attached to their child or making their child the center of their world to the exclusion of everyone else. They need to have other adults to relate to and close friends to confide in, and they need to encourage their child to do the same. Parents should never make comments like "Now that your father is gone, you are the man of the house," or "When you grow up, you can be Daddy's new wife," nor should they insinuate in any way that the child is a substitute spouse. Neither should they try to make the child feel responsible for the parent in any way or make the child feel guilty for being independent.

THE EFFECTS OF EMOTIONAL INCEST

Two of the many effects of emotional incest are chronic relationship problems and a curious blend of high and low self-esteem. In addition, when a parent becomes overly involved and overly invested in his or her child's life, problems can arise in the child's sexual development. Because the child and adult are in essence more like intimate partners than family members, it is natural for sexual feelings to arise. This sexual energy then must be dealt with, either expressed or repressed. The child may choose to express the sexuality in the form of excessive masturbation or promiscuity, or repress his or her sexuality and later pay the price of sexual dysfunction or lack of sexual desire. This is especially true if there are rigid and strict family injunctions against sex.

Being a parent's surrogate partner as a child can have a profound effect on one's life. The following are some common characteristics resulting from the silent seduction of a covertly incestuous relationship.

1. A love/hate relationship with the covertly incestuous parent
2. Emotional distance from same-sex parent
3. Guilt and confusion over personal needs
4. Feelings of inadequacy
5. Multiple relationships
6. Difficulty with commitment
7. Hasty commitments
8. Regret over past relationships
9. Sexual dysfunctions
10. Compulsions/addictions

AVOIDING EMOTIONAL INCEST

In addition to the issues I've already discussed, there are several things you can do as a parent to avoid establishing an emotionally incestuous relationship with your child, including:

✦ *Don't look to your child for emotional support.* This includes sharing personal information about yourself when the sole purpose is to unburden yourself.

✦ *Avoid putting your child in the middle between you and your spouse.* Don't share details of the problems you are having in your marriage, and most important, don't complain about your spouse (or ex-spouse) to your child.

✦ *Don't frustrate your child's natural drive toward self-sufficiency* by being overly protective or overly rigid, by discouraging friendships and ties outside the family, or by treating your child as if he or she were a lot younger than he or she is.

✦ *Encourage your child to be different from you.* Don't praise your child just when he or she does something the way you would or thinks the way you do. Make positive comments about the way your child differs from you as well.

✦ *Be a parent to your child, not a friend.* Give your child the safety and security of limits, and be prepared for the fact that your child may get angry with you.

✦ *Don't play favorites.* Many parents find themselves drawn more to one child than another. This is especially true if you were a favorite child. But you must work hard to counter this tendency by looking for and rewarding the positive qualities of each child. Try to treat all your children equally in terms of the important things like affection, rule setting, and punishment. While each child may respond differently to you and to these things, generally speaking, each child should be able to rest assured that you are going to be fair with him or her.

✦ *Make sure your child knows that you can take care of yourself.* When you are having problems, reassure her or him that you are taking the steps necessary to resolve the problem.

✦ *Make adult relationships a priority.* Set aside ample time to be alone with your spouse and/or adult friends. Go on weekend trips, go out to eat without your children, have a weekly date or a weekly lunch with a friend. In doing so you are not depriving your children as much as getting the support you need in order to be a good parent and providing a healthy model of adult life.

RESTORING A HEALTHY BALANCE

Parents often unwittingly violate the parental guidelines listed above. Most of us were not taught them, and many of us grew up with parents who modeled a less healthy way of relating to children. But it is never too late to make changes, changes that can affect your child's life significantly.

Unfortunately, it may not be enough to reinforce the boundaries between you and your child or to increase your support network. Dr. Patricia Love, in her book *The Emotional Incest Syndrome*, recommends that you also make amends to your child, especially if your child is twelve or older. Dr. Love calls this a "Realignment Session," a brief, to-the-point meeting where you explain what has happened, apologize for your actions, and describe the changes you are going to make. She suggests that if you think your child will have difficulty listening to you, write your thoughts in a letter. Dr. Love suggests the following steps:

Assure your child of your love. For example: "First of all, I want you to know that I love you and that I'm trying hard to be a good parent."

Describe your past actions. For example: "There have been many times when I didn't set limits because I didn't want you to be angry with me," or "I gave you too much information about my private life," or "I've played favorites. I've been easier on you than on your sister."

Let your child know how you feel about what you did. For example: "It's really hard for me to admit my mistakes," or "I feel guilty for putting my needs before yours." Take full responsibility for your actions. Don't let your child protect you from your feelings.

Share key information. Although you don't want to turn this into a "confession" or another time when you unburden yourself at your child's expense, you did have reasons for your actions, and hearing your explanation might help your child. For example: "After you were born, your father and I started having a lot of problems. We both tried, but somehow we couldn't resolve them. Finally, we both just stopped trying. I found it much easier to look to you to get my needs met. I now know that it was wrong to make you my friend. I taught you to take care of me instead of me taking care of you." Be careful that you don't share information that is none of the child's concern and don't let yourself off the hook.

Absolve your child of guilt. Let your child know that he or she has no reason to feel guilty, that the enmeshment is totally your responsibility. For example: "You were not responsible for the way your father treated you. I set the situation up by preferring you to him," or "It's not your fault I never date. I just don't have enough confidence in myself."

Apologize and assure your child that you no longer require his or her emotional support, and commit to a healthier relationship. For example: "I am truly sorry for what happened. I wish I could change the past, but I can't. What I can do, though, is make sure you know that you are not responsible for me or my feelings. And in the future I will be here as your parent, but not as your partner or best friend. We'll still be close, but I'll be there more for you emotionally instead of the other way around. And I'm going to spend more time with people my own age, and I want you to do the same. That doesn't mean we still won't have plenty of time together, because we will."

Emotional incest can be just as damaging to a child's sexuality and self-esteem as overt incest. By following the guidelines I have provided, you should be able to avoid this tragedy. If you need more help, refer to the "Parental Issues" section at the end of the chapter, read Dr. Patricia Love's book, *The Emotional Incest Syndrome* (see Bibliography and Recommended Reading), or seek professional help.

Sibling Sexuality

In addition to discussing the influence you as a parent have on your child's sexuality, we also need to examine the role siblings have on one another's sexual development, the importance of boundaries and privacy between siblings, and how to deal with the issue of sibling incest.

Aside from his or her parents, a child's siblings will be among his or her most important role models. A young girl may look up to her older brother, for example, and admire the way he looks, the way he dances, the way he handles himself around girls. Thus, he becomes an example of the kind of boys she will want to date. On the other hand, if her older brother constantly criticizes her, makes fun of the way she looks, bosses her around, or even hits her, she may get the idea that this is the way all boys are.

Same-sex siblings also have an effect on one another's sexual development. A good case in point is that of Charlene and her sister, Diane. Charlene was a beautiful young girl who was very popular with the boys. From the time she was in junior high, she began begging her parents to let her go out on dates. Finally, when she was a freshman in high school her parents agreed that she could double-date. Every weekend, Diane, Charlene's younger sister by two years, watched as her older sister left the house in a flurry of excitement for her dates. Diane couldn't wait until she became a freshman and was able to date and have the fun she saw her sister having.

If we stopped the story here we would have an example of how one sibling positively affected the other in terms of dating. But let's continue the story.

After about six months of dating, Charlene began to come home late from her dates, breaking her curfew more times than she kept it. Her parents became very upset and began to ground her, refusing to let her go out until she learned the rules. Thus began a seemingly endless cycle of Charlene's promising she'd be "good," only to break her curfew once again and be grounded the next weekend. Diane watched as her sister moped around the house, cried in her room, and raved and ranted about how her parents were "unfair."

Eventually, Charlene began to sneak out of the house at night to be with boys when her parents were asleep. Diane knew when she did this and wanted to tell her parents, but kept silent out of loyalty to Charlene. Finally, Charlene was brought home by the police one night. She and a boy had been cited for curfew violation. In desperation, Charlene's parents sent her to live with an aunt for the summer, hoping that some time away would calm her down.

How do you think all this affected her sister, Diane? Did she become wild like her sister when she became a teenager? Or was she so frightened of becoming like her sister that she went the other way and became a model child, one who never broke her parents' rules concerning dating? Did she think that her sister spent entirely too much time and attention on boys, to the detriment of her studies and her family? Or did she think that what her sister did was "cool"?

The point here is that we know that Charlene had some effect on Diane's perception of what dating was all about. In this particular case, Diane was so traumatized by the constant fighting that occurred between Charlene and her parents that she decided she wasn't going to date boys until she was at least a senior in high school. She turned down dates and didn't even go to the prom when she was asked in her junior year. It was far more important to Diane to please her parents and have harmony in the house than to risk displeasing them by dating.

She married a young man while in her first year of college, more because she knew her parents would approve of him than for love. Today, Diane is very unhappily married. She feels she missed out on her teen years and regrets not having dated more, and she longs for the kind of romance she imagines other women have experienced.

In addition to being role models (good and bad), siblings affect one another's sexual development in numerous other ways—by making fun of one another's looks, boyfriends, or girlfriends; by the amount of rivalry and jealousy between them; and by the kind of emotional closeness they share.

One sibling can damage the self-esteem of another by constantly teasing or criticizing her or him about how "ugly," "fat," or "stupid" she or he is and thus cause the other to believe that no one will want to date her or him. If one sibling is more attractive or popular than the other, especially if he or she lords it over the other, that too can damage the self-esteem of the one who is seemingly less attractive or popular. And, if there is constant rivalry or competition between two siblings, it can cause them to be competitive with their friends and even their lovers.

In addition, siblings often experience sexual feelings for one another. Because they are in constant contact, and because they witness each other's sexual development at the same time that they themselves are developing, it is not uncommon for siblings to feel aroused while in the other's presence. This is especially true if one or both parade around the house half-dressed or nude. Sometimes siblings will admire, make comparisons, and even engage in sexually tinged play with one another, such as tickling, teasing, or "accidentally" walking in on one another in the bathroom. These reactions are all normal and natural. Usually societal and cultural prohibitions regarding sexual activity within families ensure that these feelings will not be acted out. (Almost every known society has incest taboos that existed long before the study of genetics led humans to the realization that inbreeding was unhealthy for the species. It is assumed that these prohibitions were put into effect to protect the family unit and to ensure that people would leave their family of origin to form ties with other families, thereby strengthening the bonds in the larger community.)

Siblings frequently engage in sexual experimentation. While you naturally want to stop the behavior, do not make the event traumatic or guilt-inducing. Inform both children that under no circumstances are they to engage in any sexual activities together, that these activities are for when they are adults and are restricted to people outside of the family.

SIBLING INCEST

There are several circumstances that can occur within the family to cause siblings to break the incest taboo.

First, children who do not get what they need from their parents will often turn to one another. When children cannot depend on their parents for nurturing, affection, and encouragement, they sometimes turn to siblings and become stand-in parents to one another. A younger sibling will often look to an older one for the nurturing and guidance he or she doesn't get from their parents. This gives the older sibling far too much influence and power over the younger one, which in turn can invite sibling incest. This type of incest is often referred to as nurturance-oriented incest, and it is more erotic than abusive and can last for years.

Second, when the structure of the family breaks down because of parental conflict, drinking, drugs, violence, or emotional instability, then incest taboos are more likely to break down as well. Sometimes siblings in troubled homes seek each other out for comfort, and comfort turns to sex as mentioned above; more frequently, however, anger that cannot be expressed toward parents is often acted out on siblings. An older male sibling, seething with rage toward his parents, perhaps having been sexually abused himself, turns on a younger female sibling and sexually molests her. This type of incestuous experience is sometimes referred to as power-oriented incest.

The important thing to remember is that sibling incest is more likely to occur if there is parental neglect or abandonment, so that brothers and sisters begin to need each other for solace, nurturance, and identity, or as a vehicle to express rage and hurt.

Third, if one child witnesses or is privy to the fact that the father or stepfather is sexually abusing a sister, for example, the male sibling will often take this as permission to do the same.

Fourth, parental attitudes toward the opposite sex can also create an environment that is conducive to sibling abuse. For example, if both father and mother are misogynistic, meaning that they both have a distrust, dislike, and disregard for females and view them as inferior to males, this attitude will obviously be passed down to their children. Male children will be given preferential treatment, and female children will be regarded as inferior to the males in the household. This kind of attitude gives the message to the males that they can demand subservience from their sisters and can do whatever they want to them. Since females are not respected, the males know that their word will be honored over their sister's, and thus they do not fear punishment.

And finally, in addition to these family dynamics, children and teenagers who become sexual abusers often do so because they were sexually abused themselves, by someone inside or outside the family. Sexualized too early, full of anger and self-loathing, these victims often lash out at the weakest, most convenient person they can find—someone they know cannot or will not defend himself or herself. Males more than females tend to identify with their aggressors, meaning they become like the person who abuses them, as a way of coping with their pain and anger. But female children who have been abused can also reenact their own abuse by having power over a younger, weaker sibling.

If you discover that sibling incest is occurring within your home, it is a sign that the entire family needs professional help in the form of family therapy. If one of your children has actually become a sexual *abuser* (he or she is more than three years older than the sibling and has forced the younger one into sexual acts, inflicted physical pain, or used intimidation to get his or her way), both children need specialized psychotherapy immediately. We will discuss childhood sexual abuse further in later chapters.

Whatever happens between siblings is a reflection of what is going on in the family in general, whether it is sibling rivalry, siblings becoming too dependent upon one another, or sibling abuse.

PARENTAL ISSUES: FAMILY RELATIONSHIPS

◆

EXERCISE

Try to recall the kinds of relationships your family members had with one another. Were your parents openly affectionate with one another, or did they confine any evidence of intimacy behind closed doors? If the reverse was true, were they inappropriate in the way they showed affection toward one another, becoming too overtly sexual in the presence of their children? Did you see your father try to be affectionate with your mother only to be rebuffed with, "not in front of the children"? Or did you see your father grab at your mother's breasts or butt without showing regard for her feelings, forcing her to slap him away or retreat in embarrassment? Were you and your siblings close and affectionate with one another, or was there constant conflict? Were boundaries respected in your home?

If you are having some difficulty recalling, the following questions may help spark your memory:

1. How did your parents express their affection toward one another?
2. Were your parents ever overtly sexual with one another in front of you?
3. Was your privacy respected within the family?
4. Was there sexual energy between you and one or more of your siblings?
5. How was this handled in the family?

6. Was there ever a sexual incident between you and a sibling?
7. How did you feel about this?

————————— ◆ —————————

If your boundaries were continually violated by other family members, you will probably have problems with setting limits yourself. This can mean that you get too close to someone too fast, that you become invasive or intrusive sexually, that you become overly possessive of your lovers, or even that you have crossed the line and inappropriately acted out sexually, either by forcing others to have sex, by continually getting involved in illicit affairs, or by acting out sexually with children.

You may have had the opposite reaction and built walls around yourself to protect yourself from being hurt or intruded upon again. Intimacy and even friendship may be a problem. Wary of close love relationships and commitment, you may have compensated for being intruded upon by becoming overly protective of your emotions.

PARENTAL ISSUE: EMOTIONAL INCEST

It is important to understand that parents recreate their own family systems. Most parents are not malicious and are not aware of the effect they have on their children. What is happening is that a part of their own childhood is buried within. Sadly, if you do not take the time to see your own childhood for what it really was, the pain gets passed on from one generation to the next. You will continue to expect your children to be there for you in ways you hoped your parents would have been. When this expectation goes unmet, you will see your children as ungrateful, unloving, and ungiving. Willpower or the right set of moral standards isn't enough to produce lasting, healthy changes. Only by facing one's past can one take responsibility for oneself and reclaim the vitality surrendered by being a parent's surrogate partner.

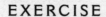

EXERCISE

Were You a Victim of Emotional Incest?

Respond to the following statements as honestly as you can, answering "yes" if you identify with it.

1. I was the source of emotional support for one of my parents.
2. I felt closer to one parent than the other.
3. I got the impression a parent did not want me to marry or move far away from home.
4. Any potential boyfriend or girlfriend was never "good enough" for one of my parents.
5. I felt I had to hold back my own needs to protect a parent.
6. I felt responsible for my parent's happiness.
7. I sometimes felt invaded by a parent.
8. One of my parents has unrealistic expectations of me.
9. One of my parents was preoccupied with drugs/alcohol, work, outside interests, or another sibling.
10. One of my parents was like my best friend.

If you answered yes to three or more of the above statements, you may have been what Dr. Patricia Love calls "the chosen child" and suffered the emotional abuse of a parent who was overly involved in your life. If this is true for you, I recommend you read her book *The Emotional Incest Syndrome*. It will tell you what you can do now to reverse the negative effects in your adult life.

As you have seen in this chapter, there is no other environment more influential to a child's sexual development than that of the home and family. This influence can be a positive one, encouraging a sense of security, confidence, and naturalness about sexuality, or it can be a negative one, exposing the child to sexual attitudes and behaviors that are inhibiting or exploitive.

The family home should be a place where a child can feel and be safe and can learn positive sexual attitudes and proper boundaries, not a place where negative, exploitive, or abusive behavior abounds.

When parents model healthy attitudes and communication skills, when affection and sexuality are seen as natural, and when privacy is respected, the home and family become a positive environment for healthy, nurturing sexuality. Take a good look at the environment you are exposing your child to daily, and work on presenting the best example you can of healthy intimacy and sexuality.

4
◆

Raising a Child with a Healthy Body Image

I f a child grows up with a good body image, that child has a head start toward growing up to be a sexually healthy adult. Providing your child with a positive body image will be one of the greatest gifts you can give her or him, one that will not only affect your child's sexuality in a powerfully positive way, but one that will affect every aspect of her or his life.

I will begin this important chapter by explaining exactly what body image is and how it relates to your child's sexuality. Body image is our view of our own physical appearance; it is the picture we have of our body—what it looks like to us and what we think it looks like to others. A positive body image is an important part of self-esteem, and having high self-esteem is vital to establishing intimacy with others. High self-esteem involves the belief that one is valuable and deserving of loving relationships and being secure enough to risk having others find out that one is not completely perfect.

Not surprisingly, the way we feel about our body directly affects how we feel about our sexuality. If we like the way our body looks, if we feel attractive physically, we will have a lot more confidence in our sexuality and our sexual attractiveness than if we don't like our body and don't feel physically attractive. This all seems rather logical, but what isn't logical is how each of us determines whether we are physically attractive or not. A person's view of him or herself has as much impact on his or her ability to form intimate, loving relationships as does that person's actual physical appearance—in some cases more.

Why is it that someone who by most people's standards would be considered extremely attractive can be as insecure about how he or she looks as someone who is far less attractive? And why is it that some people who actually have less to work with in terms of physical attributes can end up coming off as extremely attractive? And even more important, who really determines what is attractive and what is not?

Parents have by far the most influence on how their child will feel about his or her body than any other factor, as I have indicated in the following list.

A child's body image is affected most strongly by:

1. How well his or her parents like and accept their child's body.
2. How much importance his or her parents place on physical attractiveness.
3. How well his or her parents like and accept *their own* bodies.
4. Peer acceptance and rejection and how much the child's parents are able to counteract negative feedback.
5. The role of the media and how much the child's parents are able to counteract it.

PARENTAL APPROVAL OR DISAPPROVAL

Our body image comes to a great extent from the physical and emotional input we received as children. You as a parent have the most profound effect on your child's body image. If you like how your child looks and tell him or her so, your child faces the world with a head start. If, on the other hand, you dislike your child's appearance, his or her body image will be tremendously influenced in a negative way.

Kevin began to dislike his body very early on due to the fact that he knew his father disliked it.

My dad was a jock, and he wanted me to be one too. But I was more frail like my mother. He was constantly on me to gain weight and to "toughen up," as he put it; but no matter how much I ate or exercised, I remained thin with very little musculature. By the time I was in high school, I was convinced that no girl would want to date someone like me with all the jocks around, so I just never asked anyone out. It wasn't until I was in my early twenties that some girls seemed to find me attractive. Today, even though I have girlfriends, I'm always self-conscious about their seeing me with my shirt off because my chest is so underdeveloped.

THE ROLE FATHERS PLAY ON THEIR DAUGHTERS' BODY IMAGE

Fathers have a tremendous effect on their daughters' body image for several reasons. In order to develop self-assurance, a daughter needs to feel that her father thinks she is an attractive person in both body and soul. This provides the basis for her confidence as a woman and allows her to realize that she is worthwhile and that, in her future relationships with men, she should be respected.

If a girl knows that her father loves her and thinks she is attractive, she is more likely to feel attractive to other males. If, on the other hand, she feels rejected by her father or thinks he sees her as unattractive, she may generalize this to all males.

Many fathers have a difficult time when their daughters reach puberty. A father may feel proud that his little girl is growing up and at the same time want to hold on to her. Because of this internal conflict, some fathers give double messages to their daughters, such as telling them "You look so pretty" one day and "You look like a tramp" another. Still other fathers who were always very affectionate with their daughters suddenly push them away when they reach puberty and no longer show them any physical affection. This kind of behavior may cause a girl to hate the changes going on with her body and her body itself.

Unfortunately, fathers have to walk a fine line between focusing too much and too little attention on their daughters' looks and sexual development. They need to compliment their daughters and let them know they love them just the way they are, without placing too much emphasis on looks and without being seductive.

Fathers of preadolescent girls have to work hard to adjust to their daughters' budding sexual maturity and to begin the sometimes painful task of letting them go emotionally to some extent. While it is natural for a father to worry about the motives and behavior of other males, being overprotective gives the wrong message. Let your daughter know your concerns without accusing her, scaring her, or making her feel that you do not trust her. This involves not only acknowledging that she is becoming a woman, but learning to trust that she can and will take care of herself.

And while some adjustments will need to be made by a father as his daughter matures (such as no longer placing her on his lap), it will always be appropriate for him to hug and kiss her, no matter how old she is (assuming, of course, that the daughter still seems open to it).

THE AMOUNT OF IMPORTANCE PARENTS PLACE ON PHYSICAL APPEARANCE

Some parents place a great deal of importance on physical appearance, while others do not. Unfortunately, those that do tend to instill in their children an overemphasis on looks.

This was the case with Bree. Bree's mother was very pretty, and she spent a great deal of time on her appearance. By the time Bree started school, her mother had taught her to do the same. In addition, Bree's father often talked about how beautiful his wife was and how Bree looked just like her. Both parents taught their daughter that beauty is a very important thing. While you might think that Bree would grow up to have a good body image, the reverse is true. There was so much emphasis on her growing up to be a beauty like her mother that today Bree is always comparing herself unfavorably not only to her mother but to all other beautiful women. She is obsessed with her looks and cannot seem to find other things about herself that she values or believes others will value. She is also convinced that men are only attracted to a woman for her beauty and that in order to keep a man you have to work on looking good all the time.

Be careful not to place too much emphasis on physical appearance with your child. Emphasize other characteristics such as honesty, kindness, a good sense of humor, or intelligence. Even if your child is extremely attractive, in addition to admiring her looks, give her compliments on other aspects of herself, such as how considerate she is, or what a good friend she is. If she seems to be placing too much emphasis on her looks, encourage her to develop other interests and talents. And if you hear her constantly talking about the appearance of others, make comments such as, "Well, yes, she is a beautiful child, but look at the way she dances, isn't she a wonderful dancer?" or "Yes, she is pretty, but she is also smart."

THE ROLE A PARENT'S BODY IMAGE PLAYS

In addition to whether or not parents like the way their child looks and how much importance they place on physical appearance, another factor that influences a child's body image is whether her or his parents are satisfied with the way they themselves look. A parent with a poor body image can pass on negative attitudes and feelings to his or her children, causing the children to dislike their bodies. This is especially true if a child resembles a parent who dislikes her or his own looks, as did Marsha's mother:

From the earliest I can remember, my mother was always battling with her weight. She went on diets of all kinds, sometimes starving herself for days. When I reached ten years old, she started to focus on my weight as well. The doctors told her I was of normal weight and that I would grow out of my baby fat, but she didn't believe it. She started putting me on diets and paying a lot of attention to what I ate.

This continued throughout junior high school. By the time I entered high school, I had a serious problem with my self-image. I imagined I was fat and saw myself as overweight when I looked in the mirror, even though I was getting thinner and thinner. By the time I reached sixteen, I was throwing up any food I ate and had become bulimic. I have spent the past seven years overcoming my problem and working on seeing myself accurately instead of so critically.

Toni's family handled a similar situation in a completely different way. An extremely attractive woman who carries herself regally, Toni told me her story:

In my family we all have big noses, but my parents and grandparents always taught us to have pride in them because they were a mark of our ancestry. My grandparents came from Italy, and in the particular region where they were born, a big nose was a sign of the aristocracy. So I grew up liking my nose even though it is very large. I have always felt very fortunate to have been raised to have pride in the way I look because I see so many others who are always trying to change their features with plastic surgery.

Unfortunately, most parents are not like Toni's. Since many are critical of their own bodies, they are equally critical of their children's bodies.

PEER ACCEPTANCE OR REJECTION

Another factor influencing a child's body image is the amount of acceptance or rejection he or she receives from peers. A major obstacle to raising a sexually healthy child is the fact that today's children are shackled with tremendous pressure to be thin, sexy, beautiful, or handsome. Never before have children had more pressure to conform regarding their appearance, their behavior, and their sexuality.

It is very important to children and adolescents to be accepted by their peers, and those who have this acceptance tend to have high self-esteem, while those who experience rejection, teasing, or indifference tend to have lower self-esteem. Rejection or indifference from the opposite sex can be particularly devastating and can be the start of a child's believing that he or she is not attractive or desirable, as it did with Lili:

> Boys just never paid any attention to me in school. I was taller than most of them, and my parents couldn't afford to dress me very well. I was so envious of the girls who wore designer jeans and Reeboks. By the time I was in junior high, I just gave up trying to get their attention. I didn't feel like I had a chance of getting a boyfriend, so I tried to convince myself that I really didn't want one.

Name-calling is extremely hurtful to children and can affect their body image negatively. Names such as "Beanpole," "Fatso," or "Four Eyes" can stay with someone a lifetime and take a prominent place in someone's self-concept, as it did with Tom:

> It's pretty difficult to think of yourself as sexually attractive to women when you were called a nerd or a fag most of your childhood. Those words still ring in my ear every time I even think of asking a girl out.

Sometimes a child has the extra burden of having a physical characteristic or handicap that singles the child out. Some are so embarrassed by their body that it prevents them from entering a relationship at all, as it did with Jacob.

Jacob was convinced that he was too short for any girl to like him. He was so convinced of this, in fact, that he avoided asking girls out all during high school. At a recent five-year class reunion he was surprised to discover that several women had been dying to go out with him in high school, but he never asked.

COUNTERACTING NEGATIVE PEER FEEDBACK

As a parent you need not only to be understanding concerning the kinds of feedback your child is receiving about her or his body and perceived attractiveness, but to help your child cope with peer rejection, criticism, or name-calling.

One way to do this is to let your child know that almost everyone is teased and called names when they are a kid. Tell your child about your own experiences with this.

In addition, talk to your child about reinterpreting negative labels. For example, let's say that your child is hurt that her peers are making fun of her because she is taller than most other girls. Try explaining to her that many famous models are extremely tall and that many men prefer tall women. In this way you change the idea that a female's being tall is a negative.

COUNTERACTING SOCIETAL AND MEDIA MESSAGES

Yet another role parents play in determining whether their child has a positive or negative body image is whether they go along with or counter societal and media messages concerning what is attractive or unattractive.

THE ROLE OF THE MEDIA

The entertainment and advertising media not only promote certain ideals in terms of how the body should look, but often, in the absence of other sources of information, become a child's teacher of what a normal and healthy body should look like. By trying to conform to our culture's ridiculous ideals, children often place themselves in a no-win situation where they will never be satisfied with their bodies.

For example, girls tend to compare themselves with the kind of physical perfection they see on TV or in magazines, and as a result, even very attractive girls are certain that they're too fat or too thin or that something is wrong with their thighs or their breasts.

Males are also bombarded with advertisements for gyms and home exercise equipment and the constant message that females only like males who are physically fit. A boy can't help but feel bad about himself when what he constantly sees on television or in magazines is girls going crazy over a sun-tanned Adonis with a huge chest and arms.

It is vitally important that you as a parent counter the messages that your children receive from the media and explain to them that there is not one standard for beauty or attractiveness.

When your son talks about wanting to have a "great bod" like Arnold Schwarzenegger, tell him that he can certainly do this if he wants to put in the amount of time and effort it will require to accomplish that goal. But also tell him that there are a lot of other male body types that are attractive, and point some out to him. For example, show him that swimmers have very attractive bodies, as do runners. They aren't as bulky, but they are muscular in their own way. Tell him that girls like all kinds of bodies on men. Some like super-muscle-men like Schwarzenegger and Sylvester Stallone, but many prefer body types like Johnny Depp's or Brad Pitt's, and some even like nonathletic "scholarly" types. Sit down with him and help him assess his body type to see what is realistic for him. Or suggest he talk to his coach at school or even a medical doctor to get feedback on his body type.

If your teenage daughter complains that her breasts are too small, explain to her that not all men like big-breasted women.

She may just think you are trying to make her feel better, so let her know that there have been studies showing that many men actually prefer small-breasted women.

Not long ago, two Florida psychologists devised a study that examined male and female ideals about body image, using breast size for women and chest size for men. The results, published in *The Journal of Social Behavior and Personality*, show that neither sex has a correct perception of the other's ideal. Women believe than men prefer larger breasts than men actually prefer. And men believe women prefer larger pectorals than women actually prefer.

Point out to your daughter famous movie stars and models, as well as athletes, dancers, poets, and chemists who are very attractive women even though they are small-breasted. Clip pictures of attractive women with small breasts out of magazines, and then sit down with your daughter and try to discover why she is placing so much emphasis on her looks and why she is so insecure about herself. Talk about how the rest of her life is going—her schoolwork, her social life. Ask her what her dreams are for the future, what she has been focusing on lately. From this talk you may discover the reasons for her focus on her body and her negativity about her breasts.

If your daughter is concerned about her breasts being too large, follow the suggestions above (pointing out that some males like big breasts and some like small). Focus on building up her self-esteem and letting her feel good about her body the way it is. (If her breasts are abnormally large to the point of interfering with her posture, you can talk to her about eventually having breast reduction surgery.)

Countering the "Thin Is In" Message

Wanting to emulate a movie star or an athlete is nothing new for children, but the current craze is different. Today, children are getting caught up in image obsession at younger and younger ages, and for the first time, boys are almost as vulnerable to it as girls are. There seem to be two reasons for this change. First of all, kids are virtually immersed in the media, and second, their own parents are absorbed with diets, exercise, and health and nutrition reports. The net effect is that children are striving to meet standards of beauty that earlier generations of kids weren't even aware of. In a study of three hundred children conducted by Children's Hospital Medical Center of Cincinnati, twenty-nine percent of third-grade boys and thirty-nine percent of third-grade girls said they had dieted; sixty percent of sixth-grade girls and thirty-one percent of sixth-grade boys reported trying to lose weight. Another recent study found that eighty percent of fourth-grade girls were already dieting.

Body shape has become a common topic among even the very young. They spend a lot of time talking about how they think they are fat and who they think is fat. It is no surprise that eating disorders are cropping up at earlier ages. Bulimia and anorexia, once largely a problem for teenagers and college-age women, are not striking children and preteens.

What can you do to diffuse these messages?

+ Don't dwell on dieting or your own desire to lose weight. As mentioned earlier, parents' unforgiving attitudes toward their own bodies have an impact on children. Children don't understand that a parent doesn't need the calories that a child must have for growing.

+ Help your child stay in touch with his or her body. Watching television for long periods of time tends to make children more passive and less likely to develop a strong sense of their own bodies. As a result, they are more likely to live vicariously through characters they see on TV. Those children who are not in touch with their own bodies or their own activity are more susceptible to media-developed images.

+ Don't panic when your child makes an offhand comment about his or her body. Children naturally compare themselves with others. But if your child says, "I'm too fat," don't say, "You're fine as you are," and dismiss his or her concerns. Empathize while helping your child put his or her worries in perspective.

✦ Try not to comment on your child's body in ways that can be unintentionally hurtful or invasive. A statement you might think is harmless, like "You're a big kid" or "You could lose five pounds," can resonate for a child with insecurities.

✦ If your child tells you her or his pediatrician, dance teacher, or coach has made a critical remark, talk about it with her or him. Kids are extremely sensitive to perceived criticism.

✦ To minimize media influence, exert more control over your child's TV watching. But be realistic—these images are everywhere. Help your child think more critically about the images he or she sees by explaining that someone in the ad may be unhealthily thin or that there are different kinds of beauty. Try to change the question from "What's wrong with me?" to "What's wrong with this ad?"

How do you know when your child is excessively concerned about his or her body? The biggest clue is if he or she is constantly talking about the subject. If your child starts to isolate him or herself, preferring rigorous exercise or dieting to hanging out with friends, always finds a reason to skip dinner, or has a dramatically distorted view of his or her body, it may be a good idea to talk with a therapist or child psychologist.

Try to discover where your child's negative feelings come from. Often when kids talk about their bodies, they are trying to tell you something else as well.

SOCIETAL MESSAGES

We are all taught from an early age that those who are attractive are also more worthy, and we are all taught just what is considered attractive in our particular social circle. This training begins very early on when the cutest babies and toddlers are given the most attention by outsiders. Slowly, as the child grows up, he or she will be treated well or not, depending upon how cute he or she is, what kind of clothes he or she wears, and what color of skin she or he has.

Studies have shown that attractive children tend to develop more self-confidence and have higher self-esteem than those children who are perceived as less attractive. If adults smiled approvingly and told you how cute or how pretty or how handsome you were as you are growing up, you probably felt very good about your body and the way you looked. On the other hand, if insensitive adults said things like, "My, she is a fat one, isn't she?" or "He must look like his father" (implying that he doesn't look like his *attractive* mother), you probably ended up not feeling very good about your appearance at all.

One of the main reasons so many women perceive their bodies as problems is that we live in a culture that dictates that women must be beautiful to be worthwhile, and then sets up standards of female beauty that are not only impossible for most women to live up to, but are unhealthy as well. For example, many diets and all surgery to control weight are physically dangerous.

Getting and staying thin have become major pastimes for females, consuming a significant amount of their time, energy, and money. According to Judith Stein of the Fat Liberation Movement, the emphasis on thinness in our culture not only oppresses overweight women, it also serves as a form of social control for all women.

Until very recently, males have not had to suffer quite as much pressure regarding the way their bodies should look, but all that is rapidly changing. As mentioned above, today, males are constantly being pressured to work out, pump up their muscles, and stay physically fit.

You will have your work cut out for you in terms of countering societal and media messages about what is acceptable and unacceptable physically. From the time your child is a toddler all the way up to a young adult, you will need to teach a different message, one that encourages your child to value his or her body for what it gives the child (movement, protection, fun, etc.) instead of how it *looks*. For example, it is important to teach your child that one's body is a gift. Reinforce this way of thinking by commenting on how strong your child's body is, by stressing to your child all the wonderful things his or her body allows him or her to do—run, kick, jump, swim. (I will also talk about this in Chapter Eight, "Teaching Sexual Values and Responsibility.")

A child with a positive image of herself or himself, including body image, is going to grow into a confident adult who appreciates, respects, and has pride in her or his body. Parents have a tremendous effect on how a child feels about his or her body. You as a parent need to teach your children:

+ to appreciate, respect, and honor their bodies.
+ that other people will find them attractive for other reasons aside from their physical attributes.
+ to value attributes in others aside from just physical attractiveness.

PARENTAL ISSUES: YOUR BODY IMAGE

If you have a negative body image, this will influence how you view your child, whether you feel accepting or critical of your child's looks, and how much emphasis and pressure you put on your child concerning his or her looks.

The sad truth is that some of us are simply not able to appreciate our beauty no matter how much others recognize it. Often this is because as children and adolescents we felt we were ugly. In fact, research shows that the self-image we had as an adolescent tends to stay with us throughout our lifetime. That means that if you were an awkward, pimply-faced teenager who was made fun of, you probably are carrying around that picture of yourself in your mind no matter how you look today. And the reverse can be true. If you were an attractive, popular teenager, you probably tend to feel pretty good about yourself today, no matter what shape you are in. While you may be critical of the fact that you have gained weight, for example, you probably still feel better about yourself than the person who was less popular and attractive as a teenager.

WHAT ARE THE MESSAGES YOU HAVE RECEIVED CONCERNING YOUR BODY?

Because your image of yourself will so profoundly affect your child's body image, if you have problems with your body image, it is important that you discover just how this image was formed and that you work on improving it.

◆

EXERCISE

Childhood Messages

1. Make a list of all the negative messages about your body you remember receiving as a child. Include verbal and nonverbal messages from your parents and nicknames and insults from your siblings and peers.
2. Put a star beside each message that still has an effect on you (those you still believe, those that are still replayed in your head). These are the negative messages that you will need to focus on changing.
3. Now take a close look at each of these negative messages and use your logic to decide whether or not this message is accurate and applies to you today. For example, if you were teased about having acne all during your adolescence, but today have clear skin, take a good look in the mirror and acknowledge the change. You might want to say out loud to your image in the mirror, "I have clear skin now."

   If, on the other hand, you still suffer from the same problem you were criticized or teased about as a kid (you still have that birthmark, you are still short, you are still overweight), you will probably need to work on your anger at being put down for something that either you can't help or that is obviously a problem you haven't yet been able to solve. Try saying out loud to all those who put you down in the past, "You had no right to make fun of me," or "I hate you for causing me to feel so bad about myself." Releasing your anger in this way will help you avoid turning it on yourself in the form of self-criticism.

◆

EXERCISE
Messages from Lovers

In addition to parental messages or messages you received from other children when you were growing up, the feedback you've received from sexual partners has also affected your body image. With just a comment or two, a lover has the ability either to improve or damage one's body image. Because we are generally so vulnerable with our lovers, their opinions about our bodies affect us tremendously.

Even if a lover tells you lovingly that he or she wishes you would lose or gain weight, exercise more, or buy some new clothes, that message can shake your confidence. If he or she begins to nag at you continually, the damage to your body image can become more severe. And, in the heat of an argument, if a lover calls you "ugly," "a fat slob," "repulsive," or "thimble dick," you can feel cut to the very core. Not only will the insult devastate you in the moment and make it difficult for you to feel safe with that lover again, but chances are, you will replay that insult over and over in your head hundreds of times, the result being that your self-esteem will be continually whittled away.

List all the positive and negative messages you remember receiving from lovers past and present. Put a star beside every negative message you still believe. These will be the messages you need to work on changing. Follow the same instructions as in the previous exercise.

◆

HOW EMOTIONAL, PHYSICAL, AND SEXUAL ABUSE AFFECT OUR BODY IMAGE

Sometimes a person's low self-esteem and poor body image reflect the fact that something occurred in childhood to erode his or her confidence. Nothing harms a child's confidence more than experiencing emotional, physical, or sexual abuse, particularly when that abuse comes from the child's parents. When a parent abuses a child, that child will tend to blame him or herself because it is easier than experiencing the sense of alienation created by admitting anger toward the abusive parent. A great deal of this self-blame turns into self-loathing, in particular a hatred of the child's own body. In addition, many emotionally abusive parents will verbally attack the child's physical appearance.

If a child is physically or sexually abused, she or he is especially likely to have a problematic body image. Those who were physically or sexually abused as children often ignore, neglect, and even abuse their bodies since they see them as objects of shame. Survivors of abuse tend to cover up their bodies, hiding them from themselves and the rest of the world.

If you were emotionally, physically, or sexually abused as a child, you will need to be aware of the damage done to your body image. Make a list of all the messages you feel you may have received from this experience. For example: "My body is filthy," "I am used goods" (from sexual abuse), "I am so ugly no man will ever want me" (from emotional abuse).

Once again, either use your logic to help you work on recognizing that, in fact, these messages are not true, even though they felt true to you as a child, or express your anger toward the person or persons who abused you and thus caused you to have these beliefs about yourself. You can do this either by pretending to talk to him or her, or by writing a letter that you do not send. If you continue to believe the negative messages, you will need to consider therapy. Survivors of childhood abuse often need help in order to absolve themselves completely of the guilt, shame, and negative body image that the abuse caused.

YOUR SELF-PERCEPTION

For many people, their *view* of themselves has as much impact on their ability to form intimate, loving relationships as does their actual physical condition—in some cases more. We've all known people whom we consider to be especially blessed in the looks department—the gorgeous woman at work, the handsome guy who lives down the street. We usually assume that these people know they are attractive, and we even think they are probably conceited about their looks.

No matter how many times it happens, we are always shocked to discover that, often, these good-looking people are insecure or shy, or that they even feel unattractive. Time after time in television interviews, we hear beautiful movie stars tell us that they don't really feel attractive at all, and we are always surprised to hear it.

Most people have negative body images not because they have unattractive bodies, but because they see themselves inaccurately. Their images of their physical selves are distorted, either because they see their overall size and shape inaccurately (seeing themselves as much fatter, thinner, taller, or shorter than they actually are) or because they see specific body parts in a distorted way. When the latter occurs, not only do they perceive their long nose, acne, wide hips, sagging breasts, or large behinds as more grotesque than they are, but they see their imagined or real flaws dominating their entire physical selves, as Clarissa did:

> Everyone tells me that I am so pretty, but I know I'm really not. They don't know that I have these huge hips and thighs. That's because I do such a good job of hiding them. All I see when I look in the mirror are my hips and thighs. They disgust me so much that I know they would disgust other people if they saw them.

Unfortunately, Clarissa has been blinded to her other physical attributes—her beautiful skin and hair, her lovely shoulders and breasts, her striking facial features. All these beautiful parts of her are overshadowed by her dislike for her hips and thighs.

Many people are very poor judges of themselves and have a distorted view of how they impress others. Most people, especially women, are not as unattractive as they think. About one-third of Americans, particularly women, report being strongly dissatisfied with their bodies. And women are more likely to have a negative self-image than men. In fact, studies have shown that relatively few women look in a mirror without focusing on all the things they'd like to change, whereas men tend to be more accepting of what they see. Women tend to distort their perceptions of their bodies negatively, while men—just as unrealistically—distort their perceptions in a positive, self-aggrandizing way.

Almost all women have something they don't like about their body. Women put an overemphasis on the way their body looks and assume that men are attracted to them solely or primarily because of their body. They don't take into account their personality, their wit, their mind, their sensitivity, their ability to relate to others, and most important, their ability to love.

◆

EXERCISE

Getting to Know Your Body

How realistic can your body image be if you don't really know what your body looks like? Many therapists advocate standing nude in front of a full-length mirror and honestly assessing your body. But that is probably asking too much for the average person, and if you are already critical of your body, it may just reinforce your negativity. Instead, begin slowly and really concentrate on one part of your body at a time. Start with your feet. Look very closely and carefully at them, touch them, get a sense of their texture. Write down on a sheet of paper or in your journal at least two positive things about how your feet look or how they feel.

Proceed up the full length of your body, doing the same with your calves, your thighs, your hips, buttocks, genitalia, stomach, chest, arms, neck, and face. It will help tremendously if you also massage or caress each part of your body both as a way of becoming familiar with it and as a way of healing negative feelings about it.

You may need to do this exercise in several sessions. The goal is finally to look at and accept the entire body. The next step is to find a time when you are alone and undisturbed. Take off your clothes and stand naked in front of a full-length mirror. Use a hand mirror or a second full-length mirror to see your back. You may only be able to look at yourself for a few minutes at first, but gradually you will feel less threatened.

When you have been able to look at your entire body (back as well as front) without feeling repulsed or disappointed, you are ready for the next step: to begin to accept your body. Begin to let go of the need to chastise yourself for all your imperfections. Take a calm, objective, nonjudgmental look at yourself and say out loud to your reflection, "I like you just the way you are. This body is fine. This body is okay."

Now express love to each part of your body, as you would to a beloved child. Start by verbally thanking your body for being there, expressing appreciation for all it does for you. For example, thank your feet for making it possible for you to walk, and run, and dance. Thank your spine for holding you up and allowing you to bend over. Thank your breasts for giving you sexual pleasure and for allowing you to feed your baby. Thank your neck for holding up your head and allowing you to look behind you.

Learning to love your body will take time. After you are able to really look at your whole self naked in the mirror without dismay or disappointment, you will gradually begin to feel a sense of tolerance and familiarity. Eventually, with practice, you will begin to appreciate and enjoy your body for all it provides you and for its uniqueness. You don't have to change your body to feel good about yourself. You can decide to accept your body and be grateful knowing it is precious just the way it is.

◆

How your child feels about his or her body is crucial to his or her sense of self-esteem, and self-esteem is closely related to sexual adjustment. If your child thinks he or she is unattractive, the child's self-esteem as a whole will be lowered. This in turn can prevent him or her from fully enjoying sex. You as a parent play a major role in determining how your child feels about his or her body. Continue working on feeling good about your own body so that you can pass on these positive feelings to your child. And remember not to place too much emphasis on looks to the exclusion of other qualities. Self-confidence is an important part of sex appeal, but it comes from the inside out. Give your child heavy doses of encouragement and love for who she or he is as a whole person. How your child feels about herself or himself *inside* has a lot more to do with body image than how she or he actually looks.

5

♦

Raising a Sexually Safe Child

A sexually safe child. Is there such a thing in these complex, difficult, and dangerous times? In the next two chapters I will outline exactly how you can go about ensuring that your child or teen is as safe as humanly possible.

I will begin this chapter by telling you how to protect your child from child molesters. This includes learning how to spot potential child molesters, how to warn your child about them, which children are the most vulnerable to attack, and at what ages children are most likely to fall prey to a child molester.

In the second half of this chapter I will tell you how you and your teen can help prevent date/acquaintance rape by following certain specific rules about dating, and how to spot a potential rapist. In addition, I will provide guidelines for preventing stranger rape. By learning all you can about child molesters and rapists, you can help prevent child sexual abuse and rape.

At the end of this chapter I will once again address "Parental Issues," this time helping you to discover whether you may have been sexually abused yourself as a child and helping you to recognize the damage it has caused in your own life. This is a particularly important section because, as I will elaborate on later, those parents who are unaware of the fact that they were sexually abused are the parents who are *least* able to protect their children from molestation and are the *least likely* to be able to spot signs of sexual abuse in their children.

In the next chapter, "Raising an Assertive Child," I will outline specific strategies to help your child or teen take an assertive stance against inappropriate and unwanted sexual advances, whether they are from adults or peers.

It is indeed a dangerous world we live in. Child molestation, child pornography, rape, and date rape are very real and present dangers. But parents who are educated about the full extent of the dangers that face their children each day have a much better chance of being able to protect their children. It is the naive, uneducated, uninvolved parent who sets a child up to be sexually abused, exploited, or raped. Your best weapon against all forms of child sexual abuse is to be educated and in turn to educate your child.

HOW TO PREVENT CHILD SEXUAL ABUSE

The sad truth is that a child who is sexually abused faces tremendous obstacles to growing up to be sexually healthy. Therefore, one of the most significant things you can do to ensure that your child grows up to be a sexually healthy adult is to prevent her or him from being sexually abused. Can a parent do this—is it within a parent's power to protect his or her child every minute of the day? The answer is yes and no.

It is not enough to teach your child to say "No!" You must be the one to protect your child from sexual perpetrators. This means you will need to keep your eyes and ears open not only for signs of abuse in your child but for suspicious behavior in the adults and older children around you. Unfortunately, this includes members of your own family.

The National Center of Child Abuse and Neglect defines child sexual abuse as:

. . . contacts or interactions between a child and an adult when the child is being used for the sexual stimulation of the perpetrator or another person. Sexual abuse may also be committed by a person under the age of eighteen when that person is either significantly older than the victim or when the perpetrator is in the position of power or control over another child.

WHO ARE THE PERPETRATORS?

✦ About 90 percent of the time, the offenses are committed by heterosexual males, and the victims are younger females.
✦ At least 80 percent of the time the child molester is someone the child knows well and trusts, most often a relative.
✦ Most victims are abused by fathers, stepfathers, and other close relatives.

Thousands upon thousands of children are sexually abused every year by relatives, caretakers, and other children. The majority of perpetrators are relatives, most notably stepfathers, fathers, uncles, grandfathers, and older siblings, as well as mothers, grandmothers, and aunts. Having a stepfather constitutes one of the strongest risk factors, more than doubling a female's chance of being sexually molested; a stepfather is five times more likely to sexually victimize a daughter than is a natural father. The majority of child sexual abuse occurs in the home or at the hands of people known to the family. Many children are sexually abused as well by coaches, camp counselors, teachers, baby-sitters, doctors, dentists, members of the clergy—people the child trusted and cared about.

It is much easier to think of child molesters as strangers, pedophiles lurking on the edges of school yards, than to think about molestation occurring in the home. Incest may be defined as sexual relations between family members who are so closely connected by blood that marriage between them is prohibited by law. This means, for instance, brothers and sisters, first cousins, fathers and daughters, uncles and nieces, mothers and sons. Laws differ, and many states have legislated against "intrafamilial" sexual relations, including stepfathers, stepdaughters, and others who, while not connected by blood, share the *structural* relationship of a nuclear family. Sexual incidents between such people could be called "psychological" incest, and the effects can be just as traumatic as the other kind.

INCESTUOUS FATHERS OR STEPFATHERS

The incestuous father is often a hardworking, intelligent, churchgoing man, often the pillar of the community. And although he is also a deeply disturbed man, this may not be evident on the surface. Even his wife, his parents, his closest friends may not be aware of his problems.

Incestuous fathers often have strong needs for physical touch, and they often don't know how to be affectionate in nonsexual ways. Four basic types have been identified.

1. *The tyrant*—authoritarian, domineering, fear-inspiring, may use force or threat of force to make his daughter (or son) submit to him. There is also such a power imbalance, both physical and psychological, between them that resistance may seem futile—not to say disobedient. This father is likely to be extremely jealous of his daughter's boyfriends and may outlaw dating entirely. He may also severely restrict her other normal social outlets.

2. *The rationalizer*—justifies what he's doing by telling himself that he's just expressing his love for his child. He may tell himself and his daughter that he's teaching her the correct sexual procedures to help her when she goes out in the world to meet boys.

3. *The introvert*—makes the family his exclusive universe, his haven from the pressures of outside life. Often ineffectual in his social relationships, the introvert is dependent on family members for everything. And if his sexual relations with his wife deteriorate, he'll turn to his daughter to fill that function.

4. *The alcoholic*—is a dependent personality who drinks in order to give himself a false feeling of independence. Alcohol does several things: It lowers inhibitions, weakens self-control, and later serves as a convenient object of blame. As far as he is concerned, it was not his but the liquor's fault that he raped his daughter.

All four types have several characteristics in common. They tend to be men who depend upon sex either to bolster their egos, reduce tension, or make them feel loved. Their incestuous acts tend to occur at times of great stress, often when their relationship with their wife is strained. Unable to turn to their wife for sexual solace, either because of fighting, because they are experiencing impotence, or because they are punishing their wife for not giving them their way, such men will turn to their (less threatening) child. (This does not imply that the wife is in any way responsible for her husband's actions.)

When the incest is discovered, these men will almost invariably deny that it happened. If denial doesn't work, they will blame the daughter (who seduced them) or the wife (who drove them to it).

Incestuous fathers, like child molesters in general, are men who feel powerless and insignificant in the adult world. They therefore feel more comfortable with those who are weaker and more vulnerable than themselves.

Most incestuous fathers were themselves sexually abused when they were children or witnessed sexual relations between their own fathers and their sisters. They tend to have been deprived of attention and affection as children, and many ran away from home at an early age.

Warning Signs of Father-Daughter Incest

1. A mother should be concerned if she finds herself feeling jealous of her daughter. This could be a sign that she unconsciously suspects that something is going on between her daughter and her husband. Try to face and analyze these

feelings, if only for your daughter's sake. It is your duty to protect your child. Very often a mother will blame the victimized daughter for the incest when it is finally revealed. This is the ultimate betrayal for the daughter, who has a poor self-image to begin with and is already feeling guilty.

2. Be concerned if your husband or boyfriend prohibits your daughter from having male friends her age, from dating, gives her the third degree after her dates, constantly accuses her of being cheap or promiscuous, or takes an inordinate interest in her menstrual cycle.

3. A mother who works at night should be alert to the quality of the relationship that develops between her husband and her daughter. This is especially true of stepfathers and daughters. Many women sense that there's something not quite right, but they deny this feeling. Don't suppress any feelings you may have, explore them.

4. Be concerned if your husband wants to spend a lot of time alone with your daughter, frequently takes her out alone, or wants to take vacations alone with her. Find out what's happening. If your fears are confirmed, act. A call to your state's child protection agency would be a good first step. Later, the local chapter of Parents United might provide useful therapy for everyone involved. (See Appendix I.)

5. Be concerned if your daughter doesn't want to stay home alone with your husband, balks at going out with him, and resists going on family vacations.

If you sense anything like these dynamics in your family, think about what's going on, keep open the lines of communication with your child, and seek professional help.

SIBLING SEXUAL ABUSE

It is estimated that sibling incest occurs five times more frequently than parent-child incest. Few people really understand that sibling incest can indeed be the sexual abuse of one child by another. The average parent doesn't want to know that his or her children have been sexual with one another in the first place, much less that one child forced the other into it. As one mother put it, "How can I face the fact that one of my children was being held captive by another of my children in my own home?"

Still another mother reacted like this:

When my daughter told me that her brother had sexually abused her when she was a child, I was shocked. I couldn't imagine what she was talking about. Whenever I had thoughts of sexual abuse, I had always thought of an adult abusing a child. But a child abusing a child? That didn't make sense. Her brother was only a few years older than her. How could he have *forced* her to do anything? And why didn't she tell me about it?

These are common reactions to being told by one of your children that the other sexually abused her or him.

Many people find brother-sister incest less reprehensible than father-daughter incest, and certainly less than father-son, mother-son, or mother-daughter incest. If a brother and sister are about the same age and are curious about each other's sexual equipment, the resulting incest may not be traumatic to either, primarily because there is no betrayal of trust. However, the greater the age difference between siblings, the more betrayal (and trauma) will be involved. A sixteen-year-old boy who coerces his ten-year-old sister into submitting to intercourse with him is messing up that girl's life, possibly forever. There is no question of consent here, certainly not of informed consent.

We discussed sibling abuse in Chapter Three, "Sex and the Family." Here, I am focusing on how to prevent sibling sexual abuse and how to look for signs of sibling sexual abuse. For purposes of convenience I refer to the abuser as a male, but remember that older sisters have also been known to sexually abuse younger brothers.

Warning Signs of Sibling Sexual Abuse

1. An older sibling seems to take too much interest in his younger sister, does not seem to have friends his own age, and is jealous of other boys' attention to her.
2. Your younger child begs you not to leave her alone with her older sibling.
3. One of your children bullies the other (frequently hits her, makes fun of her, forces her to do things for him).
4. One of your children tends to order the other one around or to "parent" the other, perhaps because you have given him too much power and authority over her (such as leaving him "in charge" of her while you are gone).
5. You have caught your children in a bedroom together with the door closed, and they acted flustered or guilty.
6. You have caught your children together half dressed or nude.

One of these signs alone does not necessarily indicate sibling sexual abuse, but if two or more of these situations are occurring in your household, you need to keep your eyes open, explore the situation further, and seek professional help.

Most parents are not on the lookout for sexuality between their children, and they certainly would never assume that an older sibling would sexually abuse a younger one. Most instead assume that their children will observe the incest taboo and that their older children will somehow feel protective of their younger siblings. This was Jenny's experience:

Looking back on it, I realize that I was being incredibly naive. My son seemed so possessive of his younger sister, but I assumed it was because he was feeling like a typical older brother. I never imagined he felt sexual toward her, and I certainly never imagined he was molesting her. She seemed to adore him, and so I thought nothing of it when they would spend time together, even though I realize now that a normal boy his age wouldn't want to spend so much time with his younger sister. He should have been out with kids his own age.

Anna also had a lot of difficulty admitting to herself that her own son was a child molester:

I realize now that my son has never gone out with girls his age, but always with girls who are much younger than himself. His wife is ten years younger than he is. My daughter says that he married her because she is so childlike, and I guess I can see what she means. I guess he does have a real problem. My daughter is afraid he is molesting his own daughter because she is the same age as my daughter was when he began to abuse her.

Some parents are blind to their son's abusive ways because they themselves grew up in an environment where males were given preferential treatment and females were treated like second-class citizens. When they have their own children, they pass on this misogynistic legacy, as was the case with a client of mine named Candice:

My mother always preferred my brothers over me. I was taught to wait on my father and my brothers and always to do as they said. My mother basically ignored me except to depend on me to help her with the chores. My oldest brother was always a bully with me, hitting me, yelling at me, making me do whatever he wanted. When I complained to my mother about him, she would just accuse me of being rebellious and of making a big deal out of nothing. Then he started coming into my room at night after everyone was asleep and touching my body. The first time it happened I tried to stop him, but he held me down and told me that if I made any sounds he would kill me. He really scared me, and I believed he was capable of doing most anything to get his way.

After that night he came into my room every night and did whatever he wanted to me. I was afraid of him, but I also knew my mother would never believe me and would take his side if I did try to tell her.

And, of course, some parents cannot recognize even the most obvious signs of sexual abuse because they themselves were sexually abused as a child and are in deep denial about their own feelings. Rita, who had been sexually abused by both her father and her older brother, was completely blind to her own daughter's symptoms and pleas for help when her older brother began to abuse the child. Having blocked out the memory of her own abuse, Rita could not afford to see her daughter's symptoms without having to face the pain of her own long-buried secret.

As with Rita, you may have been sexually abused yourself and have no conscious memory of it. If you have *any* reason to believe this might be the case, seek professional help or join a support group for survivors of sexual abuse. Groups are especially good for those who don't have clear memories because hearing others' stories can sometimes jog your own memories. I address this issue further in the "Parental Issues" section.

Males who sexually abuse their younger sisters do so for several reasons. Some have been given silent permission to act in this way by observing the way the family functions. A boy who has seen his father emotionally, physically, or sexually abuse his mother gets the message that it is okay to be abusive to females. A boy who discovers that his father is sexually abusing his sister feels that he has the right to do so also. And mothers who allow their husbands or lovers to abuse them also give the message to their male children that it is okay to dominate and abuse females.

IS INCEST OCCURRING IN MY HOUSEHOLD?

In Chapter Three, "Sex and the Family," we discussed healthy and unhealthy conditions in the household. Even if you are certain that incest is not occurring in your family, it's important to be sure that the conditions that can *lead* to it are not present either (boundary violations, emotional incest).

The important thing is not to close your mind to the possibility of incest. Many a mother does not see evidence of incest because she is anxious *not* to see it.

The following suggestions will help you determine whether sexual abuse is occurring in your home:

1. Watch out for changes in your child's behavior. Children act out sexual traumas in various ways, including reverting to bed-wetting, having recurrent nightmares, or developing an aversion to one member of the family and not wanting to be left alone with him or her. Or, your child may develop precocious sexual behavior or suddenly start doing poorly in school after having done well in the past.

2. Know the indicators of child sexual abuse.

For sexually abused children of any age:

+ Pain in the genitals

For preschoolers:

+ Redness about the genitals
+ Infections that might be caused by venereal disease
+ Sudden sleeping problems
+ A change in eating habits
+ Uncharacteristic bed-wetting
+ Fearfulness of strangers, especially men, when there has been no such fear before
+ Any overtly sexual behavior, such as your child attempting to penetrate another child's genitals or anus with their fingers, penis, or other objects

With school-age, prepubescent children:

+ A drop in school performance
+ Marked changes in social behavior such as withdrawing
+ Uncharacteristic aggressiveness
+ Infections caused by venereal disease
+ Sudden shyness with strangers, especially men

With adolescents:

+ A drop in academic performance
+ Withdrawal from peers
+ Signs of venereal disease

+ Severe depression
+ Drug and/or alcohol abuse
+ New or unusual sexual behavior

Sexual Behavior as an Indicator of Sexual Abuse

The following is a list of behaviors parents need to pay attention to in order to detect possible sexual abuse. This list was compiled by the Sex Information and Education Council of the United States (SIECUS). If your child displays one or more of these behaviors, you may want to seek professional help in determining whether there is a need for concern and/or counseling.

1. The child focuses on sexuality to a greater extent than on other aspects of his or her environment, and/or has more sexual knowledge than similar-aged children with similar backgrounds who live in the same area. A child's sexual interests should be in balance with his or her curiosity about, and exploration of, other aspects of his or her life.

2. The child has an ongoing compulsive interest in sexual or sexually related activities and/or is more interested in engaging in sexual behaviors than in playing with friends, going to school, and doing other developmentally appropriate activities.

3. The child engages in sexual behaviors with those who are much older or younger. Most school-age children engage in sexual behaviors with children within a year or so of their age. In general, the wider the age range between children engaging in sexual behaviors, the greater the concern.

4. The child continues to ask unfamiliar children, or children who are uninterested, to engage in sexual activities. Healthy and natural sexual play usually occurs between friends and playmates.

5. The child, or a group of children, bribes or emotionally and/or physically forces another child/children of any age into sexual behaviors.

6. The child exhibits confusion or distorted ideas about the

rights of others in regard to sexual behaviors. The child may contend, "She wanted it," or "I can touch him if I want to."

7. The child tries to manipulate children or adults into touching his or her genitals or causes physical harm to his or her own or others' genitals.

8. Other children repeatedly complain about the child's sexual behaviors—especially when the child has already been spoken to by an adult.

9. The child continues to behave in sexual ways in front of adults who say "no," or the child does not seem to comprehend admonitions to curtail overt sexual behaviors in public places.

10. The child appears anxious, tense, angry, or fearful when sexual topics arise in his or her everyday life.

11. The child manifests a number of disturbing toileting behaviors: plays with or smears feces, urinates outside of the bathroom, uses excessive amounts of toilet paper, stuffs the toilet bowl to overflowing, or sniffs or steals underwear. (Please note: This does not include the normal behavior of toddlers.)

12. The child's drawings depict genitals as the predominate feature.

13. The child manually stimulates or has oral or genital contact with animals.

14. The child has painful and/or continuous erections or vaginal discharge.

If you recognize any of these behaviors in your child, don't panic. Your anxiety and discomfort will only worsen the situation for your child. Instead, seek professional help and follow the advice you are given. The sooner you deal with the problem, the sooner your child will begin to heal. The longer you wait, the more damage will be done to everyone in the family and the more difficult it will be for your child to cope and heal.

By ignoring sexual abuse, you expose your child to a life of troubled relationships, an increased risk of drug and alcohol abuse, poor psychological and social adjustment, a greater degree of mental-health problems, as well as post-traumatic stress disorder. The younger the child is when the healing begins, the more hopeful is the prognosis.

There will be more on how to help your child if she or he has been sexually abused in Chapter Seven, "What to Do If Your Child Is Sexually Abused or Your Teen Is Raped."

OUTSIDE THE HOME—PEDOPHILES AND HOW THEY OPERATE

Outside the home, your child is most in danger of being molested by a pedophile. Pedophiles are people whose primary sexual orientation is to children. Those who are attracted primarily to teenagers are sometimes called hebephiles. It has been said that it is as difficult to change the sexual orientation of a pedophile as it is to change that of a heterosexual or a homosexual.

There are far more pedophiles than you might imagine. In fact, there are so many that there exist at least two national organizations of pedophiles and hundreds of extensive underground networks, including some on the Internet. The largest and most notorious organization is called the North American Man-Boy Love Association (NAMBLA). It is made up of men who advocate adult-child sex and who seek each other out to trade information, pornographic photographs, and even victims. They circulate newsletters, and there are even several "how-to" manuals on how to pick up children.

Pedophiles are not only dangerous, but clever and determined. They know that very few adults take the time and effort to be a friend to a child and that lonely children respond to those who do. Pedophiles take the time to listen, to ingratiate themselves, to gain the child's trust.

Divorced women with young children are particularly vulnerable to the charm of a pedophile. In fact, many pedophiles marry a woman in order to gain access to her children. When the children reach a certain age, the pedophile loses interest and the marriage breaks up.

SPOTTING A PEDOPHILE

If any of the men (or women) who are in frequent contact with your child exhibit the following behaviors, you will need to be especially observant and careful.

✦ The man does not have (and as far as you know has never had) a satisfying long-term relationship with someone his own age. The more you learn about him, the more alone you realize he is.

✦ If you are dating a man who seems to take more interest in your children than in you, or you have a gut feeling that something is wrong with the way he relates to your child, trust that feeling, step back from the relationship a bit, and try to gain some objectivity before allowing the relationship to deepen.

✦ If a man without children always shows up at children's parties or hangs around playgrounds, he may have ulterior motives. Unfortunately, because this is such common behavior for pedophiles, you must assume the worst even if this means being suspicious of innocent men.

✦ If a man seems just too good to be true—he loves being with children, he volunteers to baby-sit, he wants to take them on trips—he may indeed be too good to be true.

✦ If your child suddenly has an aversion to a man whom he or she used to be fond of, find out why. Talk with your child calmly, and listen carefully.

CHILD PORNOGRAPHY

Although most pedophiles photograph their victims for their own gratification, it has been estimated that child pornography is a two-to-three-billion-dollar business worldwide and represents seven percent of the pornography sold in the United

States. Pedophiles also use pornography as a seduction lure, to convince the child that there is nothing wrong with taking off one's clothes. They may the show the child other photographs they've taken and say, "These kids have their clothes off and they like it, see, they're smiling."

Although there has been a crackdown on child pornography, stemming from a long-overdue federal law signed in 1984 outlawing all forms of pornographic exploitation of children, the child-porn network is becoming even more secretive. This makes the molester's own photos of young children even more prized. They treasure these photos as keepsakes—the children may grow up into adults, but the photographs never change.

The supply of young children for sex magazines is almost limitless. Some are abducted children who are forced to participate, some are even children of unscrupulous parents who want to make extra cash. But most are runaways who are desperate for money.

CHILD SEX RINGS

Sometimes groups of children are brought together in an organized way for the purpose of molestation and/or pornography and/or prostitution. Such rings are often made up of runaways, but some come from good homes and continue living there.

One study of forty child sex rings revealed that almost half the adult offenders used their occupation as the main access route to their victims. These rings were made up of teachers, a public-health physician, a school-bus driver, a camp counselor, a photographer, and a couple of Scout leaders. These men skillfully used peer-group pressure, competition, and a variety of rewards (both material and psychological) as inducements.

There appear to be three main types of child sex rings: solo rings (involving one molester and his private harem of children), transitional rings (a network of child molesters who start by trading photographs of children and end up trading the children themselves), and syndicated rings (a highly structured ring that recruits children, produces pornography, and delivers boy prostitutes to an extensive list of customers and is run primarily for money). All-boy rings outnumber all-girl or both-gender rings by about two to one. Boys are becoming the more likely victims of pedophiles.

The location of a solo ring will not look suspicious—it will seem to be just an ordinary house where kids come in and out a lot. The perpetrator will more than likely be a man who is looked up to by his victims and very involved in youth activities. He may use monetary inducements or alcohol to lower inhibitions and may exploit children's interest in secret clubs and forbidden activities; but the main way he influences the children will be to act as if he is deeply concerned for each child.

Transitional rings and syndicated rings usually operate in big cities and attract runaways, but parents need to be aware that they exist. They often lure children with offers of modeling or acting jobs. Warn your child that if an offer seems too good to be true, it probably is, and that, if someone approaches him or her for a modeling or acting job, to get the person's phone number and let you check out whether he or she is reputable. The child should never go with such a person (even to that person's car or van) or go alone to a photographer's studio.

Child pornography victims share many of the following characteristics:

- ✦ They are between ten and sixteen years old.
- ✦ They tend to be underachievers in school, mostly due to inattention and lack of motivation.
- ✦ They spend much of their free time in shopping malls and arcades and are often alone.
- ✦ They don't tend to come from families that instill strong moral or religious values and haven't been taught to distinguish between appropriate and inappropriate behavior.
- ✦ They may have parents who are inattentive, overworked, or irritable.
- ✦ They have low self-esteem combined with a great need for affection.

A child who has more than a few of these characteristics is particularly at risk. Sexual predators can spot and exploit such a vulnerable child.

AT WHAT AGE ARE CHILDREN MOST SUSCEPTIBLE TO SEXUAL ABUSE?

Several studies have determined that there are two age periods when children seem most vulnerable to sexual abuse. These are the period between six and seven and the period between ten and twelve. But children are vulnerable to sexual abuse at all ages, from as early as infancy to as late as eighteen.

Some studies indicate that preschoolers tend to be victimized outside the home and by men under age forty who are sometimes related to the children and sometimes not. By contrast, teenagers tend to be sexually abused at home by a father or stepfather who is between the ages of forty-one and sixty-five.

Although these findings don't suggest any specific strategies, it's useful to know where the *main* dangers lie and at which ages.

More and more I have clients coming to me who suspect that perhaps they were molested even as an infant, although they have a very difficult time believing their own feelings. Some clients describe it as an inner "knowing," while others feel it in their bodies, as body memories. Some see and feel themselves as infants and then feel a tingling in their genitals or a sharp pain in their vagina or anus, as Tabatha did:

Whenever I think of myself as an infant, I feel a sharp pain in my vaginal area. This tells me that something really did happen to me as a baby, even though I don't have a clear memory of it.

Many people do not think they were sexually abused because they feel they were old enough to consent. Unfortunately, even a teenager is not old enough to understand the ramifications of having sex with an adult, especially if that adult is a relative. The adult always has more personal and usually more physical power and is always the one responsible for the act, no matter how much the child or adolescent feels that he or she wants it.

Some victims report being abused throughout their teen years and even into adulthood. This is particularly true of girls who are abused by their brothers, as Dee was:

> I was so relieved when my brother went away to college. He had been sexually abusing me ever since I was five years old, but now it was finally going to stop. But one weekend I visited him at school, and he attacked me in his dormitory. Even though I was seventeen years old, I was still no match for him.

WHICH CHILDREN ARE MOST VULNERABLE TO SEXUAL MOLESTATION?

Although all children are at risk of being sexually abused, research has shown that some children are more vulnerable than others. For example, Dr. A. Nicholas Groth, director of the sex-offender program at the Connecticut Correctional Institution in Comers, has studied more than one thousand child molesters since 1966. He reports that unhappy children are the most vulnerable to child molesters. Those who succumb without force are often influenced by a combination of soft-talking and bribery because they are lonely or neglected. A convicted offender, when asked how he picked his child victims, reported to Groth:

> I would look at a school yard and find the child who was standing alone. The child who had thin clothes in winter. The child who was not as clean because the parents weren't taking good care of him.

RISKS FOR FEMALE CHILDREN

According to David Finkelhor, a prominent expert in the study of child sexual abuse, as listed in his book *Child Sexual Abuse*

(New York: Free Press, 1984), the risk factors for *female* children include:

Social isolation: Children who play alone and have few friends are more vulnerable, as are children who grow up in isolated areas. The physical presence of friends and neighbors acts as a deterrent to potential abusers, but even more than that, lonely children may be more susceptible to offers of attention and affection in exchange for sexual activities.

Having a stepfather, one of the strongest risk factors, more than doubling a girl's vulnerability. Apparently there is substance to the notion that stepfathers are more sexually predatory toward their stepdaughters than are natural fathers. In addition, girls with stepfathers are more likely than other girls to be victimized by *other men.* Being a stepdaughter puts a girl into contact with other sexually predatory men. Some of these men may be friends of her stepfather, men who may not feel the same kind of restraint they might if she were the *real* daughter of a friend. But paradoxically, some of these stepdaughters were victimized prior to meeting their stepfather. A mother who is dating may bring sexually opportunistic men into the home, who may have little compunction about sexually exploiting the daughter if the chance arises.

The quality of the daughter's relationship to a father, whether natural or stepfather, makes a difference in her vulnerability to abuse. When a father has particularly conservative family values, for example, believing strongly in children's obedience and in the subordination of women, a daughter is more at risk. It is also true that when a girl's father gives her little physical affection, she will have a harder time refusing the intrusions of an older man, even when she suspects them to be wrong, because she has been taught to obey and because she is starved for physical affection from a father figure.

Mothers are also very important in protecting their daughters. Girls who have lived without their natural mother are three times more vulnerable to sexual abuse than the average girl. Similarly, if a girl reports that her mother is emotionally distant, often ill, or unaffectionate, the girl is also at much higher risk. Part of the problem may be lack of adequate supervision. However, daughters whose mothers work are *not* at higher risk, so it is not simply a matter of a mother's not being around the house. It seems that daughters of absent or unavailable mothers have many unmet emotional needs that make them vulnerable. Their neediness may make them conspicuous as potential victims.

There is a connection between the oppression of wives and the victimization of daughters. Girls whose mothers are powerless may more easily fall into the victim role themselves.

Victimized girls are much more likely to have mothers who are punitive about sexual matters. Those girls whose mothers warn, scold, and punish their daughters for asking sex questions, for masturbating, and for looking at sexual pictures are more vulnerable to sexual victimization than the "typical" girl.

RISKS FOR MALE CHILDREN

Because male children are even more reluctant to report sexual abuse than female children, there are no long-term studies about the risk factors for male children. (Please note the list of the common characteristics of child pornography victims on page 118. This list applies to male children in particular.) What we do know is that there are in this country today far more males who were sexually abused as children than the experts ever imagined. For many years the figures one in every three females and one in every five males were given for the number of children who would be sexually abused by the time they reached eighteen years old. But today, with more reporting of child sexual abuse occurring than ever before, we are discovering that there may actually be as many male children who are sexually abused as female children.

The sexual abuse of male children includes everything from an adult or older child exposing himself or herself to the child, to forcible rape. It includes kissing the boy in a lingering or intimate way, masturbating in front of the child, fondling of the boy's genitals, thighs, or buttocks, forcing or coercing the boy to touch the perpetrator's genitals, performing oral sex on the boy or inducing the boy to perform oral sex on the perpetrator, forcing the perpetrator's penis or other objects into the boy's anus or forcing the boy to insert his penis or another object into the perpetrator's anus or vagina. It also includes parading around the house naked in front of the child, secretly observing the child while he bathes, undresses, or uses the rest room, or performing sexual acts in front of the boy.

While both women and gay men do sexually abuse children, the majority of all child molesters are heterosexual males. If it seems confusing to you to imagine why a heterosexual male would molest a male child, it is probably because you think of sexual abuse as being a sexual act. But experts in the field of child abuse have come to realize that it is not as much a sexual act as an act of violence. A child molester is using his or her power and authority as a weapon against a child's vulnerability and innocence. In much the same way that a rapist violates his victim out of anger toward women, a child molester violates a child out of anger toward innocence—often avenging the lost innocence of his own childhood.

OUTSMARTING MOLESTERS

Even though child molesters can be clever, cunning, and manipulative, it is possible to outsmart them. By teaching your children the following information, you can prevent them from being coaxed or manipulated into dangerous situations.

HOW TO WARN YOUR CHILDREN OF THE DANGERS WITHOUT SCARING THEM

Unfortunately, part of protecting children is warning them about the dangers. Children should certainly be taught never to get in a car with a stranger, never to wander about alone, especially in deserted areas, and to be wary of such lures as the offer of affection, candy, or money, or a request for help. Your child should be told to be aware of flattery as well, and above all, never to go anywhere without his or her parent's permission.

But warning your children will require that you go well beyond telling them not to get into a car with a stranger or not to take candy from one. Make certain that your child knows how to tell when a person may be classified as a stranger or whether or not other circumstances, such as helping a stranger look for a lost dog, are okay. For example, many molesters use the "emergency lure," telling the child that his or her house is on fire or that the child's parent is in the hospital and that the molester has been sent to pick up him or her. Some even use phoney "badges" identifying them as policemen or firemen. Make sure you make it clear who is authorized to pick up your child and who is not. Give your child a code name that only you and your child know. Tell your child that unless someone uses that code name, he or she is not to go with anyone under any circumstances.

Your child will need practice in order to understand fully how to deal with strangers in various circumstances. For example, children often feel obligated to make some verbal response to a stranger such as saying "no," when it would be best to ignore the stranger altogether and walk away.

Following are some sample situations that children may encounter with strangers. From time to time (perhaps once a month) play the "What if" game with your child, or introduce the examples into family conversations, asking, for example, "Let's see what you would do if this happened." You can start this program with most preschool children (although you probably won't offer multiple-choice answers) and continue it until you feel certain that your child fully understands what to do in any given situation. In most situations, *d* is the preferred answer and *a* is an acceptable one. I have marked these with * for acceptable, ** for preferred. If your child is having trouble, offer the correct answer, and the next time you talk, see if your child remembers.

1. Pretend you are walking down the street and a stranger asks you if you want a ride. Would you: (a) Say "no."* (b) Go with him. (c) Stop and talk to him. (d) Ignore him and keep walking.** (e) I don't know.

2. What if he asks you to go for a walk with him? Would you: (a) Say "no."* (b) Stop and talk with him. (c) Go with him. (d) Ignore him and keep walking.** (e) I don't know.

3. What if a stranger offered you money or something nice to get into his car? Would you: (a) Say "no."* (b) Stop and talk with him. (c) Go with him. (d) Ignore him and keep walking.** (e) I don't know.

4. Pretend you are walking down the street and a stranger comes up to you and tells you that he will buy you something you want if you go to the store with him. Would you: (a) Say "no."* (b) Go with him. (c) Stop and talk with him. (d) Ignore him and keep walking.** (e) I don't know.

5. Pretend you are outside and a man in a car stops near you holding a kitten so you can see it. He says, "Do you like this kitten? Come to my house, and I'll let you pick one out." Would you: (a) Say, "No thank you," and walk away.* (b) Say, "Yes! I'd like a kitten." (c) Go to his house. (d) Ignore him and walk away.** (e) I don't know.

6. Pretend you are walking down the street and a stranger in a car stops and asks for directions. Would you: (a) Ignore him and keep walking.* (b) Give him the wrong directions on purpose. (c) Tell him to ask someone else.* (d) Stand back, tell him the directions if you know them, and walk away.** (e) I don't know. (Note: Notice there are two acceptable answers and one correct one in this situation. You may not agree with answer d. If this is the case, stress answers a and c.)

7. Pretend you are at a park and have to use the bathroom. A man standing near the door says to you, "Come over here. I want to show you something." Would you: (a) Walk over to him. (b) Ignore him and go into the bathroom. (c) Tell him,

"Go away. You're bothering me." (d) Go back and tell your friends or parents.** (e) I don't know. (Note: This is a difficult one. There is no other correct answer than *d*.)

8. Pretend you are outside when a man comes up to you and says, "Have you seen a little brown dog? I've lost my dog, Max. Would you help me find him?" Would you: (a) Say, "No, I can't," and go tell your friends or parents.* (b) Say, "Okay, but just for a little while." (c) Say, "What does he look like? Maybe I've seen him." (d) Ignore him and go tell your friends or parents.** (e) I don't know.

You may not want to offer all five options at once for a very young child, but select only a few. For an older child, you may want to mix up the options so they don't predict that *a* and *d* are always the right answers.

While child abduction seems to be increasing and your children need to be warned about strangers, remember that the majority of all molesters are known and trusted family friends, neighbors, older children, coaches, teachers, clergy, doctors, and yes, relatives. How do you warn your children about people they know and still expect them to be warm and trusting?

Obviously parents want to do this in such a way as not to frighten or traumatize their children. Just as you matter-of-factly warn your children about looking both ways before crossing a street, you can warn them about protecting themselves. And remember, children do not normally become frightened of cars as a result of being warned about crossing the street without looking.

Your goal is to help your child become aware of potentially harmful situations and to give your child permission to tell you if such a situation should arise. You certainly do not want to create a distrust of all family members or all friends, and you do not want to arouse fear and anxiety over new situations or new people. Nor do you want to create a fear of sexuality or foster the attitude that sexuality always causes pain and problems.

Talking with your child in a tone that is gentle and calm will help prevent these pitfalls. Hold this conversation when you have plenty of time to talk to your child in case he or she becomes anxious or has questions requiring a long discussion. Include the following points in your discussion:

✦ Don't be alone with someone who makes you feel uncomfortable, even if it is another family member. If you must be around that person, try to have someone else with you. Otherwise, avoid the person and tell me about it.

✦ If someone is talking to you or touching you in a way you don't like or you feel uncomfortable with, tell that person so. Make your feelings known very clearly and firmly. Tell the person you will report him or her to me or the police if he or she tries anything improper. If the person continues, you may have to be rude or even call the police. If you are feeling nervous, leave at once. If the person threatens you, don't be scared. Just tell me about it, and I will protect you.

✦ Avoid going places alone. Always let me know where you are going and whom you will be with.

✦ Even if the abuse involves someone in our family, I will stand by you and help you. If you don't think I can or will help you, you have permission to go talk to someone you think can.

✦ If anyone threatens you in any way, leave. Come home immediately, and if I'm not home, lock the doors, call me or the police, and don't let anyone in the house until I, or the police, get there.

PROTECTING YOUR CHILDREN AGAINST ADULTS THEY KNOW AND TRUST

In addition to warning your child about strangers, you need to teach her or him to say "no" to those she or he knows and trusts (even if it is a relative) if that person wants to touch the child in an inappropriate way. Your child needs to know that he or she can tell you if *anyone* tries to touch him or her in ways the child doesn't like and that you will listen and believe what the child says.

1. *Teach your child about good touch/bad touch.* Children should be told that no one—stranger, neighbor, relative, or family member—has the right to touch or fondle their private parts without their permission. Your child should understand that even if it is someone he or she knows and loves, it is still not right.

You can start by teaching your child about inappropriate or bad touching and how it differs from good touching. Since you've already taught your child about breasts, vaginas, penises, testicles, and anuses, you can refer to these organs as private parts. Or, you can tell her or him that private parts are the parts that shorts or bathing suits cover.

While ideally both parents should be present, either parent is effective. These are the three most important points you want to cover:

+ *No one* has a right to touch your private parts without your permission.
+ *No one* has a right to make you touch *their* private parts.
+ Being asked to touch another person's private parts or having someone touch yours is *not* a secret you can keep. You must tell Mommy or Daddy if this happens, even if you've promised not to tell, or you've been told something awful will happen to you or someone you love if you do tell. You must tell.

Your child should know these rules by the time he or she is four years old. The important thing is that your children understand that their bodies are their own domain and that no one is allowed to touch them without their permission. Let your child know that he or she has this power over his or her own body.

It's important to be as loving and natural as you can be when talking to your child about this danger, while at the same time conveying an attitude of seriousness. And remember, children learn by repetition, so just as you repeat warnings about safety, don't hesitate to repeat this one. You can incorporate the instructions into part of a general drill:

+ "What is your address?"
+ "What's your telephone number?"
+ "What's your last name?"
+ "What telephone number do you call in an emergency?"
+ "What do you do if someone tries to touch your private parts or asks you to touch theirs?"

2. *Teach your child to tell.* If someone does try to touch your child in his or her private parts or asks him or her to touch that person's private parts, teach your child to tell. Even if he or she has broken a rule (such as going to an off-limits place or playing with a forbidden playmate), he or she must tell about it. Assure your child that he or she will not get into trouble for telling.

Generally speaking, the message to the child might be: "If someone ever touches you there or asks or forces you to touch that person, please tell us right away. Even if the person makes you promise not to tell anyone, that is a promise you should not keep. If you are threatened or forced to do things, you may have to go along with it, but even if you 'swear to God' not to tell your mother, God doesn't expect you to keep promises that hurt you. Whenever someone says, 'Don't tell your mother,' that's a good way of knowing that whatever he or she is asking you to do is wrong." Children can be told these things without being caused excessive alarm or frightened unduly.

Also, when a trusted adult begins to molest a child, he or she often does it in stages, much like a gradual seduction. If your child tells right away, he or she may prevent the worst from happening. Children can quickly detect the difference between a simple affectionate hug and a sexual advance, even though they may not be able to articulate that difference yet. All they need to tell you is that the touch made them uncomfortable.

The very nature of the power relationship between adults and children often inhibits children from telling when sexual advances are made against them. Subtle or overt threats are often made to discourage exposing the situation, or the child is sufficiently sophisticated to perceive some of the consequences: loss of family income, the breakup of the family and public shame, police or social-service intervention and subsequent court trials, the possibility of psychiatric treatment or incarceration of the perpetrator.

For this reason, it is important that you repeatedly stress to your child that his or her safety and well-being must come before any other considerations. Your child will learn this as much by your behavior and attitudes as by what you tell him or her. For example, if the child realizes that you put up with abusive treatment from your spouse because you need his paycheck to pay the bills, or if you stress in word and deed that "the family always comes first," "you can't trust anyone but the family," or "what goes on in this family is nobody else's business," the child will grow up to believe that his or her feelings and needs are not as important as keeping the family together.

3. *Teach your child that he or she has a right to refuse unwanted embraces.* Don't force your child to hug or kiss people. When you push your child to "give Aunt Martha a hug" or "kiss your Uncle Bill" when the child obviously does not feel like it, you are teaching your child that he or she must acquiesce to adults' needs rather than respect his or her own.

4. *Teach your child to say "no."* A safe child is an assertive child—a child who knows how to ask for what he or she wants, a child who can say no clearly and loudly if necessary, a child who knows his or her rights, knows that no one has a right to touch her or him where she or he doesn't want to be touched. (We will talk about how to raise an assertive child in the next chapter.)

Teach your child that he or she has a right to say "no" to unwelcome advances and that he or she should walk (or run) away, no matter how trusted, loved, or close to the family the molester is. Teach her or him that often the best protection against molestation by a trusted adult is a loud, firm, clear "No!"

5. *Listen openly and attentively to what your child has to say.* One of the most important ways of protecting your child is to listen to her or him. If an adult is making your child uncomfortable or touching her or him in ways she or he doesn't like, your child will find some way of hinting that there is something wrong. Unfortunately, parents tend to listen with only half an ear, and so they miss a lot of what their child is trying to tell them. In addition, children often communicate in hidden messages. When you do decode the message, believe your child. Children almost never make up stories about sexual abuse.

Listen openly and actively. Try to understand *exactly* what your child is saying. Decoding a child's message may not be easy at first because he or she is likely to speak elliptically about what he or she experienced. Repeat what your child has said to check if you've gotten it right. Communicate to your child verbally and nonverbally that you believe her or him, and encourage his or her efforts to talk to you.

Here are two examples, one that closes the door of communication and one that encourages the child to say what's on his or her mind:

Example #1

MARK: "Grandpa keeps bothering me."

MOTHER: "Oh, you know how he is, he likes to tease people."

MARK: "I don't like it."

MOTHER: "Nobody likes to be teased, but it's all in good fun. Now go on out and play."

Example #2

MARK: "Grandpa keeps bothering me."

MOTHER: "Grandpa is bothering you? Tell me how he is bothering you."

MARK: "He keeps touching me."

MOTHER: "He keeps touching you, and that's bothering you? Tell me how he is touching you."

MARK: "He . . . he touches me all over."

MOTHER: "He touches you all over, and that makes you uncomfortable?"

MARK: "Yes."

MOTHER: "Does he touch you in your private parts?"

MARK: "Yes."

MOTHER: "Thank you for telling me. I will make sure Grandpa never touches you like that again."

As you can see, it is important to catch the opening signal, in this case, Mark's coded statement: "Grandpa is bothering me." That, of course, could mean anything at all, so you want to listen actively and openly and keep the door open. Use the same words as the child to help you understand what he or she is trying to tell you and to let your child know you are listening. Then explore the signal to find out the feelings behind it: "Tell me how he is bothering you." That allows the hidden information to come out: "He's touching me." Now you are in the position to do something about it.

Don't overlook the possibility that sexual abuse is occurring in your home. Don't blind yourself to cues or signals your child may be trying to give you or turn a deaf ear to cries for help. You are the only one who can protect your child from this devastating crime. If you don't help her or him, you will have to live with the knowledge that you might have saved your child from pain and anguish. Again I want to remind you that if you yourself were sexually abused as a child, you may be blind to the warning signs of sexual abuse with your own child. If you don't know what to do, get help. There are child abuse hotlines in every city.

Many adult women and men who were sexually abused by a parent speak of how they feel they have actually been abused *twice:* once at the hands of the offending parent and again by the parent who refused, for whatever reason, to acknowledge that there was something terrible going on in the home. Don't let this happen in your home, to your child. Prepare your child for the possibility of dealing with sexual abuse, and be prepared to deal with it yourself.

PROTECTING YOUR CHILD FROM ABUSIVE BABY-SITTERS AND DAY CARE PROVIDERS

Thousands of children are molested by baby-sitters and other caretakers every year. In order to protect your child:

1. Hire those that you already know well and have a good feeling about.
2. If you don't know the baby-sitter, get references from previous employers. If it is a teenager who has no references, get to know the sitter's family.
3. Give your child permission to question the baby-sitter's authority. Never tell her or him, "Be sure to do what the baby-sitter tells you to do." Make sure that your child is thoroughly trained in good touch/bad touch and "private parts" concepts and that if anyone touches her or him there without permission, the child can firmly say "no."
4. Tell the baby-sitter that you don't have secrets in your house and that if anyone tries to get your child to keep a secret or not tell his or her parents something, he or she *will* tell.
5. If your baby-sitter has a boyfriend or girlfriend who wants to visit, make sure you learn all you can about that person too. Otherwise, he or she cannot visit.

Be sure to check in unexpectedly in order to get a "true picture" of the place or the person you are considering to care for your child.

Find out if a day care center does criminal background checks on its staff (many states have no such requirements). If there is no state requirement to make criminal background checks, at least find out as much as you can about the people your children will be spending their days with. That means not just the teachers, but also the aides, cooks, and other employees. Ask about them. Talk to them and get a feel for the kind of people they are.

Make sure the facility has an up-to-date license. If it's not licensed, meaning not regulated, be suspicious. Licensing does not guarantee good day care, but the absence of a license needs to be explained. (The total number of licenses revoked nationwide because of abuse of children increased tenfold since 1978 to about two hundred, and most of those cases involved sexual abuse.)

Try to find the time to spend at least one day in the center yourself. This will tell you more about the quality of care your child is receiving than all the assurances from day care operators.

PROTECT YOUR CHILD FROM MOLESTATION BY OTHER CHILDREN

There are more cases than ever of child-on-child sex abuse. Many people have a difficult time believing that children can be sexually abusive. This is partly because they know so little about childhood sexuality. For example, many don't realize that boys can get an erection and have intercourse before they reach puberty. Others have trouble discerning normal childhood sexual behavior from abusive behavior. After all, many adults have fond memories of "playing doctor" or "playing house."

There is a fine line between what children do with each other normally and what children who have been molested do to each other. Normal sexual exploration or experimentation is an information-gathering process of limited duration, in which juveniles explore, visually and tactiley, each other's bodies. Juveniles involved in normal sex play or experimentation are of similar age and size and participate on a voluntary basis.

Molestation involves differences in age and strength, threats or violence, and an emotional aftermath of anger, shame, fear, or anxiety. Child offenders seek out other children whom they can coerce, fool, bribe, or force into sexual activity with them. The sexual behaviors of these juveniles may include fondling, voyeurism, exhibitionism, oral sex, or vaginal and anal penetration with the penis or other objects. The victim is not involved in decisions about what the sexual activity will be or when it will end. Some of the victims, usually very young children and infants, suffer physical trauma from the sexual assaults.

Those who are sexualized have learned this behavior somewhere, and typically that's either through watching someone else or being victimized themselves. Many of my clients, when answering my question, "What was your first sexual experience?," will tell me about how an older sibling or older neighborhood child introduced them to sex, not realizing that in fact they had been sexually abused. Sometimes this introduction to sex was made by someone several years older than themselves, and there was a great deal of coercion occurring.

PREVENTING DATE RAPE

Rape is the fastest-rising violent crime listed in the FBI's *Uniform Crime Reports.* More than half of the rapes occur between people who have met before. These are called "date rapes" or "acquaintance rapes," phrases that have become a part of our vocabulary only in the last ten years. While the terms are new, the issue is old, although just how much date or acquaintance rape occurred in our parents' and grandparents' day we will probably never know.

Preventing rape and date rape is an important issue, and it

would not be appropriate to discuss all aspects of it in this chapter. In this section I will focus on the *safety* issues, namely how to prepare your preteen and teenage daughters for dating and socializing with men in such a way as to prevent date rape, and how to spot a potential date rapist. In the next chapter, "Raising an Assertive Child," I will address the issue of date rape and acquaintance rape further, including specific assertiveness techniques your daughter can use to help prevent date or acquaintance rape, and what to tell your son about date rape and strategies to offer him in order to avoid losing control.

WHAT TO TELL YOUR DAUGHTER ABOUT DATE RAPE

The following advice on how to avoid date or acquaintance rape is based on the experience of rape counselors and rape survivors. This advice also applies to gay males, who are raped at extremely high rates in some areas.

Rules for Avoiding Date Rape

Sit down with your daughter and discuss rules for avoiding date rape, such as the following:

1. Never take a ride with a stranger. If you meet someone at an event with friends, tell your friends you are leaving, who you are leaving with, and where you are going.
2. With new dates, drive your own car and meet the date somewhere. Insist on going to places that are public.
3. Stay away from isolated areas, even when you are with another couple or a group of people. Case histories of acquaintance rape reveal that very often couples or groups "disappeared" by prearrangement prior to the rape.
4. Stay sober. Just as it is important to stay sober in order to remain in control of your car, it is also important to remain in control of your body. You are taking a major risk if you use mood-altering chemicals when you are with strangers of unknown character. Numerous studies indicate that up

to *three-fourths* of all rapists *and* victims were using alcohol or drugs at the time of the rape. Rapists often target females who are drinking, and many deliberately plan on getting a girl drunk. Some researchers have found that seventy-five percent of their sample of college men admitted to using drugs or alcohol to get sex on a date.

5. Be especially cautious if you are in a new environment, such as being in another town or at college. Acquaintance rape frequently occurs at fraternity parties (members of the sorority/fraternity "little sisters" program on college campuses have had one of the highest rates of rape of any group).

6. Listen to your own inner voice. Acquaintance rape survivors often say they had a strange feeling about the man but did not pay attention to it.

7. Determine your sexual limits and communicate them to your date. This means telling your date just how far you are willing to go on any particular date. For example: "I don't want to do anything more than kiss." If someone goes beyond your limits or pushes you to go beyond your limits, tell them so: "No, I don't want you to touch me there." We will discuss this further in the next chapter.

8. Be definite when you refuse. Speak firmly and look the person in the eyes. Research shows that the more definite a woman's response, the more a man believes her.

9. Know that you have a right to say "no." If you are too afraid of displeasing your date, you may not speak assertively. A respectful partner will not treat you badly if you set limits. While it is natural for a partner to feel disappointed and frustrated, it is not natural for him to become angry and demeaning.

10. Be aware of situations that may be misinterpreted. For example, even though it may be practical to spend the night on his couch if you're too sleepy to drive home or if you have an early morning date, the man may not believe your "no sex" limits.

11. If you have stopped seeing someone, don't let him into your

place. A surprising number of acquaintance rapes are committed by an ex-boyfriend or ex-lover.

Learning How to Spot a Potential Rapist

Your daughter also needs to learn to recognize the behaviors common to the potential rapist, to pay attention to a man's behavior, ask others about him, listen to her inner voice, and then stay away from any man who exhibits any of the following behaviors:

Men who degrade or do not show respect for women. Men who talk negatively about women, see women as whores or to be exploited, make fun of women, or make derogatory remarks about them are more likely than others to disregard a woman's wishes and commit date rape.

Men who abuse alcohol or use drugs. Men who are out of control with alcohol or drugs are more likely to lose control sexually. Some men become violent when they drink, and many drugs elicit violent behavior. But men don't have to be drunk to be dangerous. Some men can change their behavior with only one drink, and this is a danger signal.

Men who act and talk as if they know you much better than they do, who move right into your psychological space. Such a man may sit too close to you, touch you when you tell him not to, or use his body to block your way. They may push people around to get their way. They may not listen to what a woman is saying. Such young men are dangerous.

Men who are unusually jealous, possessive, or manipulative. Men who like to control women are more likely to rape them. If you are dating someone who is abnormally jealous or possessive, checks up on you, accuses you of seeing someone else, tells you whom you should see and where you should go and what you should wear—stop seeing him. He is controlling and manipulating you and will probably do so even more as time goes by. He feels inadequate in other areas of his life and tries to make himself feel important by controlling you. It is a potentially dangerous situation, and it is not going to get better.

Men who are physically violent with you or others, even if it's "just" grabbing and pushing to get their way. Men who are loud and abusive in their behavior toward others, including other men, are trouble.

Men who are unable to handle sexual and emotional frustrations without becoming angry.

Men who don't see you as an equal, either because they are older or because they see themselves as more intelligent or socially superior to you.

In addition to learning how to spot a potential rapist, your daughter needs also to learn the following:

Recognize that men are physically turned on faster than most women. Most men become sexually stimulated very rapidly, especially young men. While young women are often content to "make out" for hours at a time, young men can become sexually frustrated by long periods of kissing and/or petting. One of the reasons why so many men complain about "mixed messages" is that most men become very aroused by visual stimuli, such as watching a beautiful young woman walk across a room. If a woman is dressed provocatively and is flirting, some men think she is sending the message that she is looking for a sex partner. For this reason, young women need to recognize that what they wear, the way they speak, and how they act all send definite messages to men that may be misinterpreted. This does not mean a man is justified in becoming sexually aggressive; it just means that young women need to know the risks. Suggest to your daughter that if she is confused as to what she might be doing or saying that sends such a message, ask a close male friend or relative.

Remember that she is in control of her sexuality. Tell your daughter that it is up to her to decide how and when she wishes to become sexually involved, and it's up to her to convey clearly to others what her thoughts and feelings are regarding sexual activity. This may mean she has to go against the crowd or be the subject of teasing in order to stand up for what she believes in. And remind her that it is her right to set and follow her own standards.

WHAT TO TELL YOUR SON ABOUT DATE RAPE

It would be tragic if your son ended up raping a girl when it could have been prevented. The entire way that dating is set up has built-in problems. Boys get the message that they are supposed to be aggressive, while girls are supposed to be passively resistant and then gradually acquiesce. To add to the problems, many males often confuse sex with a competitive sport—thus the tendency to talk about "scoring" with a girl.

And look at the role the media takes in shaping the lives of our boys and girls. Many of the most popular male stars are those who portray violent, aggressive men who disrespect women, such as Sly Stallone, Clint Eastwood, and Arnold Schwarzenegger.

Men who rape are men who like to dominate and control, tend to be extremely jealous and possessive, do not respect or listen to women, and tend to be heavy drinkers. They tend to make assumptions about what a man's rights are just because he paid for the date, and they believe that their sexual urges are uncontrollable. They also tend to believe that women enjoy sexual violence and to see women as being responsible for preventing rape. Every parent of both girls and boys needs to work to counter these negative messages about the sexes and the endorsement of the "macho" personality.

Fathers should teach their sons that real men treat women

as equals. Show your son by example: Treat your wife with respect and teach him to do the same. Never stand by and allow him to humiliate his mother or sister.

In order to eliminate the crime of rape, men must become active and vocal in advocating the right of women to refuse sexual intercourse, and they must realize that any time a woman is forced to have sex against her will, it is rape. Fathers need to make this clear to their sons, their daughters, and to speak out with their male peers. In addition, sharing the following information with your son will also help to combat rape:

1. *Learn to communicate clearly with females.* If you feel a girl is sending a mixed message (flirting and dressing provocatively, but fending off your sexual advances) ask her exactly what message she really wants to send. Don't play guessing games or assume you know what the girl wants. Spend some time talking to girls about their point of view.

2. *Realize that women respond differently to sexual arousal than men.* Most women do not experience the immediate physical arousal that men do. Sexual arousal seems to take more time in women and is often triggered by different stimuli than in men. Because of this, many women are not aware that men get aroused by the way they dress or by dancing, for example. You need to be honest with women and let them know when you are becoming aroused so that they can modify their behavior if they choose to.

3. *Show respect when a woman says no.* No one likes to be rejected, but by the same token, no one has the right to force his will on anyone else. If a girl says no, try not to take it personally as a rejection, but as a message that she just isn't ready to have sex. She may care about you very much, but have other reasons for not wanting to have sex at this time. If you pressure her into having sex, you may destroy the feelings she has for you. If a woman says "no," back off and show her that

you respect her feelings. Give her time to get to know you better.

If you force yourself on a girl, you will lose her respect and trust, and you may end up in jail. It is not worth facing yourself in the mirror, or her hatred and fear the next time she sees you. Remember, word travels fast, especially on campus. If you become known as a guy who doesn't know how to take no for an answer, you'll have a difficult time getting dates.

4. *Avoid telling jokes that degrade or humiliate women.* Just as it makes you feel angry or embarrassed to hear jokes that put down your race, religion, or masculinity, jokes that degrade women or call attention to their bodies are humiliating to women. The use of sexual slang is derogatory, and using it will make you look insensitive and unkind.

5. *Stand up to your friends when they degrade or humiliate women.* The biggest influence on men is their male peers. Men have to be the ones to convince other men that women are to be treated and respected as equals. When you are with a group of guys who are talking crudely about women, don't laugh. Speak up and say, "I don't think that's funny," or walk away or in some way indicate your disapproval. Disrespectful, demeaning talk perpetuates abusive behavior toward women. Play your part in convincing men that their masculinity does not depend on putting down women.

6. *Defend a woman's right to speak assertively.* Speak out against date rape and all other forms of violence against women. Tell your buddies that you admire a woman who knows what she wants and isn't afraid to say so. Be respectful and supportive when a woman is assertive, and encourage her to voice her opinions. Women need to know that there are men who care about what they feel and think, who will treat them as intelligent equals, who are not threatened by a woman who can speak her mind.

7. *Avoid women who pose a temptation to you.* Healthy men can control their sexual urges. It is not normal for a man to lose control of himself. If you feel you have little control over your urges, you may benefit from counseling. To gain some immediate control over your impulses, avoid women who trigger them. If you feel yourself losing control, leave the situation at once. If you cannot rely on yourself to do this, ask a friend to help. You will be showing strength by leaving a potentially dangerous situation, whereas staying and forcing someone to satisfy your urges only shows weakness. Real power comes from controlling yourself, not someone else.

8. *Do not abuse alcohol or use drugs.* If you find that you lose control more easily when you are drinking or high, don't drink or do drugs. Blaming your loss of self-control on drinking is a weak excuse. One of the most important aspects of growing up lies in learning your limits. Learn how much is too much for you. Friends can help you learn at what point you are "out of it."

Don't risk harming someone else because you are too drunk to control yourself. For the rest of your life you'll have to live with the knowledge that you raped someone. If drinking makes you feel powerful, work on having power over your drinking. If you want to conquer something, conquer your drinking.

9. *Never use force to get your way.* Forcing someone to have sex is never acceptable, even with someone you know. By resorting to the use of force with a woman, you show that you are weak, unable to take no for an answer, not strong enough to control your own body, not masculine enough to walk away.

Date rape is a crime. When you force a woman to have sex, you risk facing arrest, jail time, AIDS, or other sexually transmitted diseases. You become responsible for the probable emotional breakdown of another human being. You become a criminal, whether you are ever prosecuted or not.

PREVENTING STRANGER RAPE

Make certain that your daughter follows the guidelines listed below whenever she is alone, either inside or outside of the house. (These guidelines are actually applicable for male children as well, and for adults for that matter.)

At Home

+ Always keep your doors and windows locked.
+ Refuse to admit into your home or apartment anyone whom you do not know or were not expecting.
+ Do not allow strangers to use your phone.
+ If a repairman, a utility person, or a policeman comes to the door always ask through either a partially opened, chained door or peephole to see the proper identification.
+ Leave the door open if a properly identified repairman enters, and plan where you will go if the situation becomes threatening.
+ Have the key ready before you approach your home or your car.
+ Have adequate lighting at all doors.

In the Car

+ Keep your car, tires, and so on, in good condition to prevent a breakdown.
+ Keep your doors locked at all times.
+ Travel on well-lighted streets where people are always around.
+ Stay in the car if it should break down.
+ Keep a quarter taped to a card with a tow truck number so you can pass it through a slightly opened window to anyone who stops to help.
+ Check the rearview mirror occasionally and know where to find the police, fire station, or other safe place if you are followed.
+ Sound the horn if you need assistance.

✦ Try to park your car where it is well lighted at night.

✦ Look inside before unlocking your door.

In Public Places

✦ Walk near the street and avoid places such as alleys, doorways, or shrubbery where someone could hide.

✦ Walk with your head up and with confidence; make it clear you know where you are going.

✦ Whenever possible at night, leave shopping centers, work, or public places with other people.

✦ If a driver pulls over to ask directions, call out to him or her briefly from a safe distance away.

✦ Do not hitchhike under any circumstances.

✦ Do not walk alone at night.

✦ Carry a whistle, a buzzer, or a loud siren for attracting attention in an emergency.

✦ If a car approaches you and the driver threatens you, scream and run in the opposite direction from the car.

✦ If you find yourself on an elevator with someone who seems risky, get off at the next floor. If such a person enters an elevator that you are planning to enter, wait for the next elevator.

✦ If you are harassed by a person in a public place such as a bar, report him to the owner, bouncer, or bartender.

Take the time to sit down with your daughter and devise a plan for how to handle a situation of someone attempting to rape her, including what she should do if she cannot escape. Plan whom she should notify and what hospital she should check into. Hopefully, this information will never be used, but it will give both of you a feeling of security.

By taking the steps outlined in this chapter, you are doing the very best you can to prevent child molestation and rape and to ensure that your child will grow up to be a child who looks forward to a happy, healthy sex life.

PARENTAL ISSUES: WERE YOU SEXUALLY ABUSED?

Many of you reading this book were sexually abused your-selves as children and some of you may have read my previous books, *The Right to Innocence, Partners in Recovery,* and *Families in Recovery.* Those of you who know you were sexually abused also know that your children are more likely to be sexually abused than other children.

But many of you reading the book are unaware that you were sexually abused as a child. Parents who were sexually abused themselves as children, particularly those who are in denial about that abuse (either because they "blocked it out" of their memory or have minimized its effects), are far more likely not to notice the warning signs of sexual abuse in their own children. In addition, parents who were sexually abused as children will have certain attitudes and beliefs that will profoundly affect their children's sexual development.

In addition to the fact that many people have blocked out the memory of sexual abuse, many blame themselves for the abuse, or think they were too young or too old for it to be considered sexual abuse. And there are other reasons why people are confused as to whether or not their particular experience was actually child sexual abuse—most notably the idea that unless intercourse took place, it was not sexual abuse. But many forms of sexual abuse do not involve intercourse or any kind of penetration.

Below is an abbreviated version of a list that originally appeared in *Handbook of Clinical Intervention in Child Sexual Abuse,* by Suzanne M. Sgroi, M.D. (Lexington Books, 1982). The list contains many types of sexual abuse toward children of either sex. Look over the list carefully to see if any of these things happened to you as a child.

1. *Nudity.* The adult parades around the house in front of all or some of the family members.
2. *Disrobing.* The adult disrobes in front of the child, generally when the child and the adult are alone.

3. *Genital exposure.* The adult exposes his or her genitals to the child.
4. *Observation of the child.* The adult surreptitiously or overtly watches the child undress, bathe, excrete, or urinate.
5. *Kissing.* The adult kisses the child in a lingering or intimate way.
6. *Fondling.* The adult fondles the child's breasts, abdomen, genital area, inner thighs, or buttocks. The child may similarly fondle the adult at his or her request.
7. *Masturbation.* The adult masturbates while the child observes; the adult observes the child masturbating; the adult and child masturbate each other (mutual masturbation).
8. *Fellatio.* The adult places his or her mouth on the penis of the male child or has the child fellate the male adult.
9. *Cunnilingus.* The adult places his or her mouth and tongue on the vulva or in the vaginal area of the female child or has the child place mouth and tongue on the vulva or in the vaginal area of the adult female.
10. *Digital (finger) penetration of the anus or rectal opening.* Perpetrators may also thrust objects such as a crayon or pencil inside.
11. *Penile penetration of the anus or rectal opening.*
12. *Digital (finger) penetration of the vagina.* Inanimate objects may also be inserted.
13. *"Dry intercourse."* A slang term describing an interaction in which the adult rubs his penis against the child's genital-rectal area or inner thighs or buttocks.
14. *Penile penetration of the vagina.*

If any of the above-listed acts took place in your infancy, childhood, or adolescence with someone older and you felt uncomfortable or strange about it, then you were sexually abused. Of equal importance is any indirect or direct sexual suggestion made by an adult toward a child. This is called "approach behavior." It can include sexual looks, innuendos, or suggestive gestures. Even if the adult never engaged in touching or took any overt sexual action, the child picks up these projected sexual feelings.

Keep in mind that the *intention* of the adult or older child while engaging in some of the acts (nudity, disrobing, observation of the child) will determine whether the act is actually sexually abusive. If an adult watches a child bathe, for example, but does so in a *nonsexual* way that does not upset the child, it may not be sexually abusive. But if the adult becomes sexually aroused while watching, it is then sexual abuse.

Pornography often plays a part in child sexual abuse, with the perpetrator using it to introduce the child to the idea of sex.

Another common misconception is that sexual contact with a child doesn't really cause any damage to the child as long as there is no violence or pain. While the list above seems to increase in severity, all types of sexual abuse, even inappropriate nudity and kissing, can be emotionally and psychologically damaging to a child for a lifetime, even if it is not violent, overly physical, or repeated. There is always damage and pain, even if it is emotional rather than physical, and much of this damage is caused by the betrayal by someone the child trusted and cared about. Children need time to be children before they are capable of handling any sexual relationship. Sexuality foisted upon them too early amounts to abuse, and it is still abuse even in the complete absence of physical pain.

Tad, an adult male client, told me his experience of being introduced to sex at an early age:

> I was five years old, and my female baby-sitter showed me her breasts one day. She asked me if I'd like to touch them. I didn't really, but she seemed to get mad that I didn't want to, so I did. They felt soft, but I was very uncomfortable. I knew we weren't supposed to be doing this. Then she told me to pull out my penis so she could touch it. I really didn't want to do this, but again, I was afraid she'd get mad at me, so I did it. She started rubbing it, and it felt really good, but I was really scared.

After that, I didn't really want to have her baby-sit for me again. I tried to talk my parents out of going places, but I couldn't really tell them why I didn't want her to baby-sit. I think she baby-sat for me for several years, but I'm not sure. She continued to touch me and have me touch her, but I think I have blocked out other things she did. I don't have any memory of those years with her, so I can only assume she must have abused me further. God knows what she did to me. All I know is that I have both a tremendous fear and a sick attraction to being around domineering women and being controlled sexually by them.

If you suspect that perhaps you were sexually abused, or if you already know you were and are concerned about how this will affect your child's sexuality, I recommend you join a support group for survivors of sexual abuse or even a group for parents who were sexually abused. Please refer to the last chapter of the book, "Final Thoughts," for referral sources and how to find an appropriate support group.

HOW SEXUAL ABUSE AFFECTS YOUR SEXUAL ATTITUDES AND BELIEFS

Those who were sexually abused tend to develop negative, false, or distorted attitudes and beliefs about sex. Some survivors are aware of these attitudes, but most are unaware since many of these attitudes are unconscious. One of the primary attitudinal problems with survivors is that they have a difficult time separating abusive sex from healthy sex. This is due to the fact that sexual abuse and its perpetrators teach its victims an abusive way of thinking about sex. Sexual abuse teaches its victims the following attitudes:

- ✦ In sex, there is always a victim and a victimizer.
- ✦ Sex is dirty, bad.
- ✦ Sex is something to be endured.
- ✦ Sex is something you do in exchange for something else.
- ✦ Sex is secretive.

+ Sexual desires must always be acted out.
+ Sexual energy is uncontrollable.
+ Sex is power.
+ Sex is used as a way to control others.
+ Sex is a right that men can demand of women.
+ Sex is humiliating.
+ Sex is dangerous.
+ Sex is a game.
+ Sex is addictive.
+ Sex is a way to escape painful emotions.

If you have many of these beliefs, you will need to work extra hard not to pass them on to your children.

6

$\blacklozenge$

Raising an Assertive Child

WHY ASSERTIVENESS TRAINING FOR KIDS?

In the previous chapter we briefly discussed the idea of teaching your child to say "no" to unwanted sexual advances. But teaching your child to say "no" will do very little good if he or she is unable to do so out of fear, intimidation, or lack of assertiveness. In this chapter we will focus on how to raise an assertive child, one who will not be as likely to allow anyone—stranger or relative, child or adult—to impose on him or her sexually, one who will not hesitate to say "No!" loudly and clearly, and one who will not be afraid to tell and keep telling.

(It must be understood, however, that a child is no match for an adult, and that sometimes, no matter what the child does, no matter how assertive he or she is or how loudly he or she protests, the child will be abused anyway. A child should never be led to believe that he or she is invincible and that just by being assertive, he or she can ward off a molester's advances. Neither should a child be made to feel ashamed if he or she is unable to do so. This is particularly the case with male children. Males in our culture, even male children, are made to feel that they should be able to defend themselves in order to be manly. This is a significant reason why males who are sexually abused tend to keep the molestation a secret. They are ashamed that they were not able to fight the molester off and in so doing "be a man."

In this chapter we will also discuss how to raise an assertive preteen or teen. In addition to being still at risk of molestation by adults and older children, preteens and teens are also in danger of being raped by dates or strangers. Teens need to learn assertiveness techniques to avoid these dangers.

Teens and preteens also need to learn how to set their limits and communicate them effectively in order to avoid getting involved sexually before they are emotionally prepared to do so. Part of a young girl's education should be to prepare her for the fact that boys will pressure her sexually and to let her know what she can say and do when she is pressured. Boys, on the other hand, need to be raised to respect a girl's right to say no and to understand that "no" means "no," regardless of when or why a girl says it.

Assertiveness also plays an important part in helping preteens and teens to ward off peer pressure concerning everything from taking drugs to becoming involved in sexual activities they really do not want to be involved in. In addition to all that we discussed in the previous chapter, other important factors influencing how safe a child will be are: whether he or she is perceived by others as assertive or passive, how much importance he or she places on other people's opinion of her or him, and how much he or she can withstand pressure and coercion. These are all affected by how self-confident and how assertive your child is.

Assertiveness is also an important tool for learning how to deal with sexual harassment. Today, many preteens and teens are getting jobs to help earn extra money, and many are running into situations where they are sexually harassed by fellow employees or by bosses. They need to know about this problem ahead of time and learn how best to handle it.

Last, but certainly not least, both children and teens need

to learn to be assertive rather than aggressive when attempting to get their needs met. This is particularly true for males, who, in our culture, often feel they have the right to take what they want instead of being concerned about the rights of others. While there certainly are boys who are nonassertive and girls who are too aggressive, males in our culture generally need to focus on becoming less aggressive and girls need to focus on being less passive.

Whether it is learning to say "no" assertively to a would-be molester, learning how to withstand peer pressure, or learning to state their sexual limits when they begin to date, both children and adolescents need to learn assertive behavior.

Unassertive children allow adults and older children to cajole them into sexual activities for which they are too young, too inexperienced, or ill equipped to cope. Unassertive teenage girls are unable to say "no" to the advances of teenage boys, either because they want to please them, are afraid of losing their attention, or fear angering them. Unassertive teenage boys are unable to ask out those girls they are attracted to. Aggressive teenage boys often cajole, manipulate, or even force girls into having sex with them with no regard for the girls' feelings or rights.

WHAT EXACTLY IS ASSERTIVENESS?

Assertive behavior is the balance between *nonassertiveness* at one extreme and *aggressiveness* at the other. "Assertive" should never be confused with aggressive. The intent of assertive behavior is to communicate honestly and directly, while the intent of aggressive behavior is to dominate, to get your way at the expense of others. The intent of nonassertive behavior is to avoid conflict altogether, which usually means subordinating your wishes to those of others. When we are aggressive, we are insensitive to others' rights, and we express ourselves in ways that demean, humiliate, or coerce them. When we are nonassertive, we either don't tell others what we want and think, or we try to get what we want through devious means. We let others choose for us and infringe on our rights. Nonassertive behavior usually comes from feeling helpless and threatened and makes us natural victims for aggressive people. When we are assertive we make choices for ourselves without harming or being harmed by others.

Assertive behavior is when you stand up for your rights and say directly what you believe, want, and feel. Assertive people do this appropriately and honestly while respecting other people's rights as well. The assertive person speaks up in her or his own defense, but does so without the intention of harming or putting down another person.

An assertive child is one who knows his or her rights concerning privacy and his or her body, when and how to say "no" clearly and definitely, how to run away, and to tell and keep telling until someone listens.

An assertive child grows into an assertive adolescent, who feels confident enough to ask out those he or she finds attractive. An assertive teen is one who knows his or her sexual limits, is able to communicate those limits clearly and succinctly, and is able to restate those limits over and over if need be, no matter how much peer pressure or coercion he or she may receive. An assertive female teen feels confident enough to say "no" to unwanted sexual advances, and an assertive male teen is confident enough to ask for what he wants without being aggressive and to respect the response he receives.

An assertive teen grows up to be an assertive adult, who knows how to ask for what he or she wants, both sexually and in other ways, and does not put up with behavior that is uncomfortable, unhealthy, or abusive.

HOW WELL DO YOU MODEL ASSERTIVENESS?

As I've stated over and over, you have a tremendous influence on your child, especially as a role model. If you are an assertive person, both in your dealings with your partner and with your children, your child or teen will learn to be assertive from your example. On the other hand, your children will also watch and learn from you when you act nonassertively or aggressively and will learn those behaviors as well. In addition, you affect just how assertive your child or teen will be in the future by how assertive you allow your children to be with you now. The following checklist will help you discover both how assertive you are with your children and how much you allow your children to be assertive with you.

+ In most situations, does your child understand exactly what you expect from him or her? Are your requests specific as to time, place, and other requirements?

+ Do you demand only what your child can realistically complete at one time?

+ When you make requests of your child, do you provide follow-through help?

+ Do you respect your child's privacy and personal rights (such as allowing privacy in her or his own room)?

+ Do you allow your child some autonomy, or do you feel threatened with the unknown or when you are not in direct control (such as always having to know whom your child is talking to on the phone)?

+ Do you set realistic limits for your child (curfew, TV time and content, chores)?

+ Do you encourage your child to handle some situations independently but with your support (allowing him or her to resolve difficulties with friends; helping, not doing his or her homework)?

+ Do you encourage your child to stand up for his or her rights with others as well as with you?

+ Do you allow your child to disagree openly with your judgment (such as allowing your child to choose his or her own friends)?

+ Do you listen to your child's point of view?

+ Does your point of view always have to prevail, or do you let your child sometimes "win"?

+ When you are unable to control your child, do you resort to threats, yelling, or physical punishment?

✦ Do you overprotect your child (such as not wanting her or
   him to get involved with a sport for fear of injury)?
✦ Do you allow your child to make decisions on his or her own
   sometimes (such as which dress to wear to an important
   event, which present to buy for a relative)?
✦ Do you allow your child to state how he or she feels, instead
   of telling your child how you think he or she feels?

Your answers to this checklist point out which areas of child-
rearing you could handle in a more assertive, possibly less controlling way. (Please refer to the "Parental Issues" section at
the end of the chapter for a discussion on how and why you
became so controlling.) On the other hand, if you often feel
put upon by your children, it may be a sign that you are not
acting assertively with them and are not allowing them to learn
to act assertively themselves.

You can see how these questions directly relate to how assertive your child will be with peers and, later on, with partners
of the opposite sex.

The first step in learning to behave assertively with your
child is to recognize her or him as someone with certain personal rights. While it is true that you have to make some decisions for your child's welfare, you can also help her or him to
be assertive and to stand up for her or himself.

Start by observing what your child actually does and what
you expect her or him to do. This usually means distinguishing
between appropriate child behaviors and adult behaviors. Do
you sometimes expect your child to behave as an adult rather
than as a child? Part of helping your child to be assertive is to
try to avoid expecting her or him to function as an adult. Instead, your child needs you to provide support and guidance
when it is called for and needs you to allow her or him to tackle
other situations on her or his own.

TEACHING YOUR CHILD TO BE ASSERTIVE

A lot goes into teaching a child to be assertive. It involves
teaching your child how to communicate in an assertive man-

ner and raising him or her in such a way as to nurture the child's self-esteem so he or she will be confident enough to be assertive. It also involves teaching your older child that he or she has rights when it comes to his or her body and sexuality.

STEP ONE: GIVE YOUR CHILD WORDS TO SAY AND THE CONFIDENCE TO SAY THEM

It is not enough simply to encourage children to be assertive. Sometimes we have to give them words to say, at least in the beginning. Then, with practice, they can make the words their own and come up with their own way of saying what they need to say. This will require encouragement from you all along the way. Each time you hear your child being assertive, compliment her or him, tell the child how strong he or she sounds, and when you hear the child being nonassertive, gently suggest another way of saying the same thing in a more assertive way.

✦ Give your child examples of when it's okay to say "no." Be specific so that your child really understands that he or she is in charge of his or her own body, no matter what the circumstances. For example, some children are victims of other children's excessive curiosity. Prepare your child for this situation by stating: "You can tell any of your friends 'no' if you don't want them to touch or kiss you. Your body is yours to protect and take care of."

✦ Draw on reports in the media and ask your child what he or she would say or do in a specific situation, or how he or she thinks another child might handle a similar problem.

✦ Role-play or rehearse various common life situations with your child. For example, you pretend to be a stranger asking your child to help her or him find a lost animal, and see what your child does. If your child responds in an unsafe way, try it again, this time reversing roles with you playing the part of your child while he or she plays the stranger. Keep switching roles until your child is appropriately assertive.

Then give your child compliments on his or her assertive behavior.

Teach Your Child How to Make I-Statements

The best way for your child to state that he or she needs something or to assert his or her right to something is to speak clearly and in a straightforward manner. The simplest tool for doing this is called the "I-statement." These expressions not only say what you think, but also stress how you feel.

This is how to make an I-statement: Think of what you really feel (anger, irritation, guilt, jealousy, embarrassment, fear, disappointment, discomfort). Now plug the emotion into one of these sentences:

"I *feel* _____ when you do that."
"I'm _____" (mentioning the feeling).

"I'm uncomfortable" is a good all-purpose statement to describe what you are feeling. You can say you're uncomfortable when you can't pinpoint your exact feelings, but you feel a need to speak up anyway. The statement can be used in many situations without having to give reasons.

I-statements increase the odds of getting your feelings across successfully to another person. Although it may seem like a big risk to lay our feelings open in this way, if we can't say how we feel, we are a lot more vulnerable to things that will happen later if we don't speak up.

Nurture Your Child's Self-Esteem

The second part of Step One addresses the issue of self-esteem. In order for your child to be assertive, he or she must have self-confidence and high self-esteem. Self-esteem is how we feel about ourselves, our overall judgment of ourselves. Our self-esteem may be high or low, depending on how much we like and approve of ourselves. If we have high self-esteem, we have an appreciation of the full extent of our personality.

This means that we accept ourselves for who we are, with both our good qualities and our so-called bad ones. If we have high self-esteem, it can be assumed that we have self-respect, self-love, and feelings of self-worth.

Your child's overall self-esteem is affected by a number of things: most importantly, the amount of nurturing, attention, and caring the child receives, especially during the first few years of his or her life; the amount of encouragement the child receives when he or she attempts something new and the kind of feedback the child receives for his or her endeavors; the amount of acceptance or rejection the child receives from parents, siblings, teachers, and peers; and the child's success or failure in school, in sports, and in social interactions.

Those who were treated with loving kindness and respect by caretakers and others around them generally have a much higher sense of self-esteem than those who were neglected or abused as children. Likewise, those who were encouraged by others end up feeling much better about themselves than those who were criticized or discouraged in other ways.

Nothing is as important to our psychological well-being as our self-esteem. The level of our self-esteem affects virtually every aspect of our lives. It affects how we perceive ourselves and others, and it affects how others perceive us and subsequently how they treat us. It affects all our choices in life, from what career we choose to whom we choose to get involved with. It affects our ability to take action when things need to be changed and our ability to be creative. It affects our stability, and it even affects whether we are followers or leaders. It only stands to reason that the level of our self-esteem, the way we feel about ourselves in general, would affect our sexuality and our ability to form intimate relationships.

In addition, self-confidence is one of the strongest skills that a child or adolescent can have when dealing with peer pressure. Those young people who are unsure of themselves and need acceptance by peers to validate who they are, are more likely to give in to negative peer pressure than those who have developed a good self-concept. Self-confident teens are much less likely to be flattered or frightened into doing something they are not ready for.

All the issues we have addressed thus far—bonding, nurturing, and touch; parental messages; family relationships; body image; protection from abuse and exploitation—are all important components in raising a child to have high self-esteem.

In addition, it is vital that you are able to distinguish between your child's behavior and your child herself or himself. Suppose your child does something that you have forbidden, like telling a lie. While it is important for you to enforce appropriate discipline, it is crucial that you not withdraw your love and reject your child because he or she was "bad." Your child must feel that whatever his or her transgression, he or she is still loved and valued. While the behavior itself may be "bad," he or she needs to know that he or she is not a bad person; the child's sense of worth and acceptance needs to be maintained. If you withhold love as a punishment, your child will come to feel unloved and unlovable.

In Part II we will look further at the connection between self-esteem and sexuality. In my book *Raising Your Sexual Self-Esteem* I have written about sexual self-esteem extensively. You may also want to refer to the classic book *Your Child's Self-Esteem* by Dorothy Corkville Briggs (see Bibliography and Recommended Reading) for further information on how to encourage high self-esteem in your child.

STEP TWO: TEACH YOUR CHILD OR TEEN THAT HE OR SHE HAS SEXUAL RIGHTS

Older children need to know that each of us has certain sexual rights. The following list of sexual rights was adapted from the book *Talking Back to Sexual Pressures* by Elizabeth Powell. Go over the list with your older child (age eight and up) and explain each right to her or him, answering her or his questions as you go along. This provides you an excellent opportunity to explain such things as obscene phone calls and sexual harassment and to clarify issues like sexual advances made by professionals such as teachers, doctors, dentists, and the clergy.

1. No one has the right to touch you in any way unless you give your verbal permission.

2. You have a right to be protected from any contact or experience with an adult when the purpose is to sexually arouse or sexually satisfy the adult.

3. You have a right to refuse any type of sexual contact at any time or any place, regardless of how sexually aroused the other person is.

4. You have a right not to be talked to in a sexual way by anyone unless you give your permission.

5. No teacher, minister, doctor, psychologist, or any other professional has a right to pressure you into sex or make sexual suggestions or advances toward you.

6. You have a right to use the telephone without being harassed by obscene phone calls (uninvited sexual remarks or sexual threats).

7. You have a right to work at your place of employment without sexual communication or sexual contact of any kind, especially when this talk or contact is intended either to threaten your job or as a promise to better working conditions. This kind of behavior is called sexual harassment, and it is against the law.

Sexual harassment ranges from unwanted sexual comments made at inappropriate times (often in the guise of humor) to coerced sexual relations. It includes any and all of the following behaviors:

+ Verbal harassment or abuse
+ Subtle pressure for sexual activity
+ Sexist remarks about a person's clothing, body, or sexual activities
+ Leering or ogling of a person's body
+ Unnecessary touching, patting, or pinching
+ Constant brushing against a person's body
+ Demanding sexual favors accompanied by implied or overt threats concerning one's job or student status
+ Physical assault

8. You have a right to wear the clothing of your choice, providing it is within the law. Just because you wear something that someone else considers "sexy," it does not mean that person has the right to harass you or make unwanted sexual advances toward you.

9. You have a right to know the intentions of a partner before you have sexual intercourse.

10. You have a right to know if a potential sex partner has a contagious disease of any kind, or could possibly have been exposed to one.

11. You have a right to insist that a sexual partner wear a contraceptive or other protective device before engaging in intercourse.

ASSERTIVENESS FOR TEENS

Teenagers can protect themselves in several ways by being assertive:

+ They can decrease, or completely eliminate, their risk of contracting a sexually transmitted disease or STD (by insisting on using condoms every time they have sex).

+ They can decrease their risk of pregnancy or of impregnating someone (by insisting on wearing and using protection).

+ They can decrease their risk of being raped by an acquaintance (by being able to say "no" firmly and loudly).

+ They can decrease their risk of being sexually harassed (by knowing what to say in response or by reporting this behavior to those in authority).

For years, assertiveness classes were primarily taught to *females*. But both male and female teens need to learn assertiveness. Both males and females need to know how to deflect sexual pressure, and both need to know what to say to help themselves in a variety of sexual situations.

For example, males are also vulnerable to sexually transmitted diseases; they can impregnate someone with whom they never would have had sex if they had been thinking rationally; and they can be sexually pressured by both male and female employers. Fifteen percent of the males in the federal work force claim to have been sexually harassed on the job.

College counselors report that a surprising number of men are reporting that they are worried about sexual pressure from women. They feel it is so unacceptable to refuse a woman that if they don't want to go as far as their partners do, they become anxious and concerned about their sexuality.

TEACHING YOUR TEEN ASSERTIVE BEHAVIOR

The following assertiveness guidelines are provided so that you can teach them to your teen or have your teen read them directly out of the book.

Learn to speak assertively. In order to speak assertively, you must know what you want. Practice being clear and assertive about the messages you send. Don't assume that others know what you are talking about. If you are not sure whether other people understand your position clearly, ask them what they think you said. This will give you an idea how you come across to others.

Make sure you speak loudly and clearly. Keep your message short and direct. Don't end your sentences by asking a question. If you say "no," don't give a lot of explanation. Understand that you have a right to say "no." Once you've said it, stick with it and don't vacillate. If you need to, repeat your message, exactly as you first said it. If you are not getting your message across, don't hesitate to call the police.

Say what you mean, exactly what you mean. If you don't mean it, don't say it. Males become confused and angry with females who they think are "leading them on." Girls need to watch the way they flirt. Innocent flirtation is one thing, but if you become overtly seductive, you need to be prepared for the consequences. Don't say "no," and then later on say, "Well, maybe," or "I'm not sure." This kind of communication gives the impression that you don't know how to make up your mind and are therefore an easy target for manipulation and coercion.

Use assertive body language. When you want to deliver a serious message, when you want to be taken seriously, look serious. Don't smile, giggle, or look apologetic. Look the person straight in the eye. Don't look away or look down. If you are saying "no," say it with your whole body. Stand tall and erect, and place your hands directly in front of you as a barrier to reinforce what you are saying. If you are not getting the results you want, do not stay and try to explain, plead, or argue. Turn around and leave at once.

Learn how to defend yourself. Unfortunately, no matter how assertive you become, no matter how careful you are, you may find yourself in a situation where you need to protect or defend yourself against an attack. For this reason it is important that you learn some basic defense techniques. Take a self-defense class, such as the ones offered by local organizations, rape-crisis hotlines, or schools.

HELPING PRETEENS AND TEENS TO POSTPONE SEX

Oftentimes teenagers become involved sexually even though they really do not intend to. Both sexes can get pressured into it, either by their dates or by peer pressure, and both can get carried away in the heat of passion. Both males and females need to learn strategies they can use to help them avoid acting impulsively.

Teach your preteen or teen that there is a continuum of physical acts in human relationships. Learning to be intimate in a sexual relationship takes time and requires a willingness to take risks. Obviously, those risks should be taken slowly and carefully and even systematically—not haphazardly. This means taking a sexual or emotional risk when it is appropriate to how vulnerable it makes you feel at that stage of the relationship. Intimacy is often established one step at a time by taking a risk, then stepping back and giving yourself some time before you take another. Below is an example of the kind of continuum a healthy sexual relationship might follow:

1. Holding hands as you get to know one another by sharing your likes, dislikes, goals, and dreams.
2. Kissing as you begin to feel safe with one another and as you continue to get to know one another.
3. Deep kissing and petting as you begin to learn more about each other physically and to know each other's moods over time.
4. More and more intimate sexual sharing as your sense of safety with the other person grows along with your sexual attraction for one another.
5. Sexual intercourse (or a comparable act) after a discussion of one another's romantic and sexual histories, including the important issues of sexual fidelity and protection against AIDS.
6. Mutual exploration of one another's bodies as you continue to share one another's histories, including the sharing of sexual and other secrets.
7. More and more intimate forms of sexual sharing as a gradual deepening of the relationship occurs and time is given to getting to know one another's personality needs.
8. A commitment to one another that may include a promise of monogamy as each discovers that he or she does not wish to be with any other person and as each discovers that he or she can indeed trust the other with his or her body, history, secrets, and most important, emotions.

Encourage your teen to become clear about what his or her "sexual policy" is and to state this clearly to his or her dating partners. Explain to your teen that because people in our society have an amazing variety of sexual attitudes and beliefs, from believing that premarital sex is wrong to thinking of sex as a form of recreation, no one can assume anything about your sexual beliefs and standards (your "sexual policy"). For this reason, experts on sexually transmitted disease and acquaintance rape recommend that teens and adults alike need to let those they date know where they stand concerning sex.

Kissing and touching someone you are attracted to causes most people to become sexually aroused, and that person will more than likely know by your response that you are aroused. Your partner needs to know what that arousal means and how far you will go with it. It is far better to say, "I do not *plan* to go further" or "I don't *intend* to go further," rather than to say, "I don't *want* to go further" or "I don't *feel like* going further"—because you may in fact want to, physically. It will probably help your partner to understand that while your body seems to want to go further, your mind has decided something else. This may sound like a small difference, but in fact it is a significant one. Numerous surveys show that men who rape acquaintances often believe she meant "yes" even though she said "no" because of the way her body was responding. Passion is not the same as intention, and you need to make this very clear.

Encourage your teen to determine what his or her particular stopping point is in any given relationship. He or she will then need to be able to communicate this to his or her partner before they get to this point. Young people need to know that saying "no" can involve physical communication: removing a hand, moving away, pushing away, restraining. However, most physical communication needs to be reinforced by verbal communication. Parents can help young people by teaching them simple verbal assertiveness techniques for saying "no."

TEACHING ASSERTIVE DATING BEHAVIOR

What Girls Need to Know

If a young woman lacks directness and assertiveness, the young men she is dating may feel she is sending them a mixed message. Men are less likely than women to recognize subtle or nonverbal sexual refusals. There is a great deal of research to back up the fact that men frequently misread women's signals, and this adds to the idea many men have that women don't know what they want. In addition, being polite at any cost can put a woman in danger.

Marion Howard, an Emory University professor who ran a "teen services" clinic at Grady Memorial Hospital, found that simply providing teenagers with information about sex was not effective in changing sexual behavior. Something was missing. So she asked one thousand sexually active girls who'd come to the clinic: What sort of help *weren't* they getting? An astounding eighty-four percent wanted to learn "how to say 'no' without hurting the other person's feelings."

1. The very first step in saying "no" is simply to *say "no" and keep repeating it*. It is important that parents tell their daughter she doesn't have to make excuses or give a list of reasons. She can just say "no":

"No, I don't want to do that."

"No. I don't *have* to tell you why. I can just tell you 'no.' "

"No. That's all there is to it. No."

"No. I've decided I don't wish to do that."

This strategy involves asserting one's rights. Most often, if the girl keeps saying "no" and says it firmly enough, the other person will accept her decision.

2. However, parents can also help the young woman understand that occasionally there are people who are so self-concerned about getting what they want that they won't listen. In such a case, the parent can help the daughter understand that another communication step can be taken. *The pressure can be turned around*. One way is to question the other person about the pressure:

"Why are you trying to make me do something after I've told you I don't want to do it?"

"Why do you keep pressuring me when I've told you 'no'?"

"Don't you believe I have the right to decide for myself?"

"Don't you respect me enough to let me make my own decision?"

"But I've told you 'no.' I'm not going to do that. Didn't you hear what I said?"

Another way is to turn the pressure around by telling the other person how his continued pressure makes the young woman feel:

"The fact that you keep pressuring me when I've told you 'no' makes me angry with you."

"The fact that you keep trying to make me do something I don't want to do makes me think you really don't care about me and just want to use me."

"The fact that you keep trying after I've said 'no' makes me wonder if I should go out with you again."

This strategy involves negotiating for mutual change. In all relationships there are conflicting desires and needs. Good relationships involve communication that makes it clear to the other person how one feels and how important the issue is to the person. Often, people truly interested in maintaining a good relationship will respond to such negotiation and stop the pressure.

3. If all else fails, however, young women need to know they have a right to *get out of the situation* by refusing to discuss the matter any more, or by physically removing themselves:

"If you don't stop, I'm going to go inside the house."

"Apparently you haven't heard what I've been saying. I'm leaving."

"That's it. Take me home."

This last strategy involves a demand for change. It is the strongest of the three strategies. Its very use signals that there is a problem in the relationship.

The pressure to go further than the girl wants often comes from a boyfriend. Because the girl may feel ambivalent about how to respond, it is important for parents to help their daughters acknowledge that ambivalence and to let them know that it is all right and normal to have such feelings. Knowing they have conflicted feelings, however, does not mean they have to act in the wrong manner. They can still say "no":

"Sure, I've wondered what it would be like, but I'm not going to do it."

"If I were going to have sex with anyone, it would be with you—but I'm not going to do it."

Of course, your daughter needs to know that sometimes a boy won't take "no" for an answer no matter how assertive she is. Refer back to the section "Preventing Date Rape" in Chapter 5.

What Boys Need to Know

Boys need to be taught to be assertive instead of aggressive. Unfortunately, even today we tend to expect our men and boys to be tough and aggressive and our girls to be sweet and passive. Boys are socialized into aggression with statements like "Be a tough guy!" and "Big boys don't cry," while girls are rewarded for being polite and are discouraged from communicating assertively for fear of being criticized as "unladylike." Boys are encouraged to "stand up for themselves," even if it means using force, while girls are taught to be reasonable and diplomatic and to try to "work things out." Girls are also encouraged to avoid violence and resolve conflict. The result is that young boys assume a power-assertive style of interacting, in which they back up direct demands with force. Because of this style, girls grow up sensing and often directly experiencing an element of fear in their interactions with boys and men.

Teach your son that a mature person is capable of and willing to try to understand another person's point of view. Even though he may not agree with it or feels disappointed, if a girl says "no," he should accept her limits. If he cannot do this, he needs to tell her that he is not interested in waiting and therefore needs to end the relationship so he can pursue one where the girl wishes to go further. He should not do this as a manipulation however, but as an honest statement of his intentions and his needs.

An immature person, on the other hand, has trouble understanding another person's sexual rights. Like a child, that person "wants what he wants when he wants it." He will do anything to get what he wants, including trying to manipulate others with lines and threats. When the other person refuses, he becomes furious or rejecting.

A mature person has the ability to postpone gratification. He knows there will always be another time and he doesn't want to make the other person feel bad about herself for simply asserting her rights.

Males in our society are brainwashed to believe they have no self-control and that they cannot turn down sex. But neither one of these things is true. Male children need to be educated about what a tremendous put-down it is to portray males as sexually out-of-control. It is not complimentary to be seen as a person who is just barely under control. This implies that men are not trustworthy and can't be held responsible, making them little more than animals when it comes to their sexual urges. The phrase "men are dogs" is a tremendous put-down of the men in our culture, even though everyone seems to laugh and think it's funny.

1. Teach your son to ask for what he wants clearly and directly. This doesn't mean that he needs to impose himself on others, force others to do his bidding, or try to coerce or manipulate others into doing what he wants. Explain to him that using "lines" is manipulative and dishonest, whereas saying the same thing sincerely is not manipulative.

2. Teach your son that an assertive person is secure and strong enough to take "no" for an answer. Remind him that just because one woman says "no" doesn't mean that he is unattractive, unlovable, or not sexy enough. And remind him that if one woman says "no," another will say "yes." There is always another time.

3. Teach your son to have enough self-respect only to want to be with women who want to be with him.

4. Teach your son that a real man can decide whether it's

wise to have sex with a particular partner. Encourage him to base his decision on the reality of the situation and not on the advice of his buddies or his locker-room pals.

5. Help your son think up assertive responses to risky sexual propositions such as:

SHE: I really want to have sex with you.

HE: I'm attracted to you, you know I am. But I'm just not ready to get involved right now.

SHE: What's the matter, you're not afraid, are you?

HE: No, it's just that this is an important decision. I don't want to be pushed into doing anything until I'm ready.

SHE: What's wrong, do you have some kind of sexual problem?

HE: No, just because I want to make my own choices doesn't mean there's something wrong with me.

6. Help your son learn to assert himself when other males pressure him into being more sexual than he wants to be. Assure him that his self-esteem should not depend on what his buddies think, that a mature man doesn't conduct his sex life for the approval of his buddies, and that a "real man" doesn't give others that much power over him.

7. Offer your son some suggestions as to how to ward off put-downs by other men.

A: What's wrong with you, don't you like sex?

B: Sure I do, but I just don't like to talk about it all the time.

8. Teach your son that he doesn't have to give in to pressure to brag about sexual conquests.

A: Who was that "ho" I saw you with?

B: Her name is Janice, and she's no "ho."

C: Man, she was fine. Are you getting your share?

B: I don't like to talk about that. It's private.

9. Teach your son what to do when a woman says "no" but seems to be saying "yes" with her body. Explain that he must be very direct with his partner even if she is giving him a double message.

SHE: No, I can't . . .

HE: (Looks at her directly) I keep feeling that you want to keep going even though you are saying "no." I don't want to do anything you really don't want to do.

SHE: I just don't want you to think less of me.

HE: I won't think less of you, but I need to know what you really want to do.

10. And last, but certainly not least, teach your son that there may always be those who put him down or tease him for defending women. Teach him that often people criticize us when they are threatened, envious, or just because they want to go along with the crowd. Sometimes it only takes one person standing up for what he believes in to make a real change. On the other hand, there may not be any obvious change in his peers' behavior, but at least your son will feel good about himself.

Sometimes no matter how assertive your child is, she or he may still be molested or raped. But this does not mean that he or she shouldn't continue working on being assertive. In fact, your child will need to work doubly hard on becoming sexually assertive. This is true for several reasons.

1. Unless they practice assertiveness, victimized children often grow up to be victimized adults, continuously allowing others to manipulate and abuse them further.

2. Those who have been sexually victimized need to be assertive not only with strangers but with sexual partners of their choice. They need to be clear about exactly what kind of touch and what kind of sexual activities they prefer so they don't end up feeling abused later by their partners.

3. Unless they become more assertive they may choose not

to become involved in sexual relationships at all. They may be so fearful of being victimized again that they shy away from future involvement.

Assertiveness can also help heal the damage caused by sexual molestation or rape. In the next chapter we will discuss how this works, as well as what else you can do to help your child or teen heal from sexual victimization.

PARENTAL ISSUE: ARE YOU ASSERTIVE, NONASSERTIVE, OR AGGRESSIVE?

As I have stated many times, you are a model for your child, the person your child is most likely to emulate. If you want to have an assertive child, you must model assertiveness.

Characteristics of *nonassertive* behavior include not expressing your own feelings, needs, and ideas; ignoring your own rights; and allowing others to infringe on them. This behavior is usually emotionally dishonest, indirect, inhibited, and self-denying. The nonassertive person allows others to choose for him or her and often ends up feeling anxious and disappointed with him or herself at the time and possibly angry and resentful later.

We do this to avoid unpleasant and risky situations, to steer clear of confrontation and conflict. The problem with this non-assertive behavior is that we usually don't get what we need, our anger builds up, and we don't feel good about ourselves.

Characteristics of *aggressive* behavior include expressing your feelings, needs, and ideas at the expense of others; standing up for your own rights but ignoring the rights of others, trying to dominate, even humiliate them. True, this behavior is expressive, but it is usually defensive, hostile, and self-defeating. The aggressive person tries to make choices for herself or himself and for others, and she or he usually ends up feeling angry, self-righteous, and possibly guilty later.

Aggressive behavior is a way of venting your anger, and

sometimes you achieve your goals, at least in the short run. The problem is that you distance yourself from other people and can end up feeling frustrated, bitter, and alone.

Characteristics of *assertive* behavior include expressing your feelings, needs, and ideas and standing up for your legitimate rights in ways that don't violate the rights of others. This behavior is usually emotionally honest, direct, expressive, and self-enhancing. The assertive person makes her or his own choices, is usually confident, and feels good about herself or himself, both while he or she is being assertive and later.

The assertive person usually achieves his or her goals, and even when he or she doesn't, the assertive person still feels good about herself or himself, knowing that he or she has been straightforward. Acting assertively reinforces his or her good feelings about herself or himself, improves his or her self-confidence, and leads to freer, more honest relationships with others.

◆

EXERCISE

How Did You Get This Way?

The way we approach relationships as adults was strongly influenced by our interactions with our own parents and other authority figures. Your nonassertive or aggressive patterns may have been planted and reinforced early on in your childhood.

One way to become aware of how you may have learned to be nonassertive is to examine the messages—explicit and implicit—that you received from your parents or other significant people in your childhood who told you how to behave. Since much nonassertiveness is an attempt to avoid conflict, a recognition of how your family taught you to deal with conflict may be useful. Some questions to consider are:

1. How did your family handle conflict?
2. How did your parents train you to deal with conflict? What were their messages? ("Don't rock the boat," "Nice girls don't argue/talk back," "Be pleasant or go to your room.")
3. Did they give your brothers/sisters the same message?
4. How do you deal with conflict now?
5. In what ways did you learn to get what you wanted without asking for it directly?
6. How do you still use those ways today to get what you want?

◆

EXERCISE

Sexual Assertiveness

Pick a time when you are feeling fairly secure and confident to do this exercise. Ask your partner for something you want or for a specific change in your sex life. Examples might be a certain kind of touch, a massage, sex at a different time of the day. Don't start with the change you want the most or something that you know your partner will have a difficult time with. Work your way up to that after a few more successful experiences of asking. It's perfectly okay to tell your partner you are nervous about asking for your needs to be met.

Although it is fine for you to ask for something without immediately having to give back, you may want to give your partner the opportunity to be assertive as well by asking him or her if there is anything he or she would like to change in your sexual relationship or if there is something he or she would like you to do.

◆

Unless you practice becoming more assertive yourself, you will pass on nonassertive or aggressive behavior patterns to your child. Work toward becoming a shining example of how assertive living can help you have a healthy and happy sexual life.

Assertiveness can help prevent child molestation, rape, sexual harassment, STDs, and unwanted pregnancy. Encourage your child, whether girl or boy, to practice the behavior and assertiveness techniques outlined in this chapter.

7

♦

What to Do If Your Child Is Sexually Abused or Your Teen Is Raped

I f your child is sexually molested or your teen is raped, it does not mean that she or he has completely lost all chance of becoming a sexually healthy adult. What it does mean, however, is that you and your child will need time to heal and will probably need professional help. In addition, your child or teen will need your loving support and assistance.

IF YOUR CHILD HAS BEEN SEXUALLY ABUSED

If your child informs you that he or she has been sexually molested, there are several things you can do to help alleviate his or her suffering. First (and this will be difficult), try to control your own anxiety level. If your child senses that you are completely devastated by the situation, it could magnify his or her own reaction. While it is perfectly okay for you to let your child know that you are hurt or angry, try to stay focused on your child's reactions rather than getting totally caught up in your own (at least when you are in your child's presence).

Second, while it is entirely understandable for you to be in shock and to have a difficult time believing that such a horrible thing could possibly have happened to your child, for your child's sake, don't allow yourself to stay in disbelief and denial. As hard as it is for children to tell their parents that they were abused (and it is extremely difficult), can you imagine how they feel when they are not even believed?

Children seldom lie about being sexually abused. Very young children don't have the vocabulary or the concepts with which to construct such a fabrication. Children who keep changing their story often do so either to protect the molester (especially if he or she is someone they love, like their father) or because the molester has threatened to kill them, their parents, other family members, or a pet. Those few cases (and they are few) in which a child has been known to lie are usually cases in which the child has been used as a pawn in ugly divorce and child custody cases. So whatever your child tells you, believe her or him.

Third, make certain that you don't blame your child in any way or even *imply* blame. Parents should never say things like "Why did you let him do it?" or "Why didn't you run away?" Such questions imply that the incident was somehow the child's fault. It is always the responsibility of the molester. No matter how "seductive" or "flirtatious" a child might seem, he or she is not to be blamed for an adult's inability to control his or her impulses.

Perhaps most important of all, comfort your child. Let your child know that you still love and value her or him. Your child will continue to be fearful for a time afterward and will need a great deal of reassurance concerning his or her worth, safety, and acceptance in the family. In a very important sense, how your child ultimately responds to the trauma, and how badly her or his self-esteem is affected, depends largely on how your family responds to the situation. The best book for parents on the subject is *The Silent Children: A Parent's Guide to the Prevention of Child Sexual Abuse*, by Lynn Sanford. (See Bibliography and Recommended Reading.)

Once in the open, the situation must be handled sensitively for your child's sake; interviews, medical examinations, and court procedures must be conducted with your child's feelings in mind.

In most situations, it is important to bring your child in for a thorough medical examination. Injuries will be treated and evaluated, all bodily orifices will be examined for injuries, and a test for venereal disease will be administered. There is a sensitive chapter on this subject in the book *Your Children Should Know*, by Flora Colao and Tamar Hosansky. They note that medical procedures tend to be frightening to young children, especially those who have been sexually abused. They suggest that the doctor should talk to both parent and child, in language the child can understand, about what's going on.

Pelvic and anal examinations are uncomfortable at any time, but after a sexual assault they are usually extremely painful. In addition, the child is often in the same physical position as when he or she was assaulted.

Be aware that most physicians are required to report sexual assaults on children to the police. This means that child protective services or your local police will undoubtedly contact you for more information. You will need to prepare your child to be interviewed when they contact you. Even if the molester is a relative, it is vitally important that you encourage your child to tell the truth about what happened. Nothing will be gained if you or your child try to protect the molester. That person needs help in order to stop this damaging behavior. If he or she does not get help or is not stopped, he or she will continue to molest your child and other children.

Even if the incident is not reported by your physician for some reason, you need to report the molester yourself to the police or the child protective services in your area. The most important reason for this is to protect your child and other children from future molestation, but it is perfectly understandable for you to also want punishment for the molester, especially if it is someone outside of the family. To report this, call your local police, or child protective services listed in your phone directory, or by calling Child Help U.S.A. (See Appendix I.)

When the offender is a relative, it is often much more difficult to make a report. But the only way your family is going to heal is if the entire family receives help. And often, as mentioned above, the only way to get a molester to stop is to report him or her. Child-abuse hot lines and special counseling centers now exist in every state. They offer support, counseling, referrals, and legal assistance to victims as well as victimizers.

WHAT ARE THE EFFECTS OF CHILD SEXUAL ABUSE?

Since the offender is almost always someone who has been in a position of trust with regard to the child, the main long-term effect of sexual abuse is to make it very difficult for the child to trust anyone completely ever again. Without immediate and intensive therapy, your child will probably never regain that ability to trust and so may avoid intimate relationships entirely or enter into unhealthy or abusive relationships.

Not only has your child been deprived of his or her sexual innocence, but he or she has been deprived of childhood as well. Most abused children will miss certain important developmental steps, so even when the abuse ends, they find they don't feel like other children and they don't know how to feel close to people. It's typical for a child who's been molested to become emotionally retarded or fixated at the age when the molestation began. For example, if it started at five and was discovered at nine, we may find that emotionally she or he is still back at five.

Another dangerous aftereffect has to do with the premature sexualization of the child. As mentioned earlier, many victimized children may start acting out seductive and sexualized forms of behavior (such as introducing other children to sexual activities that he or she learned from the molester).

There is also the danger that as your child grows to adulthood (or earlier), he or she may try to gain control over what happened to him or her by acting it out with younger, smaller, or more vulnerable people than him or herself. The child may, in other words, become a child molester too.

There are many other effects of child sexual abuse. Refer back to Chapter Five under the "Parental Issues" section for a list of long-term effects of child sexual abuse.

Some of the many long-term symptoms that victims of child sexual abuse suffer as adults are specifically focused around their ability to function sexually.

✦ Lack of sexual desire or inhibition of sexual feelings; inability to have an orgasm.

✦ Sexual dysfunctions such as vaginismus (an involuntary contraction of the vaginal muscles, making penetration difficult or impossible) and painful intercourse.

✦ Inability to enjoy certain types of sexuality (can't be penetrated but can engage in oral sex; can't be fondled but can be penetrated; can't be touched in certain parts of the body).

✦ Problems with sexual identity.

✦ Promiscuity (continuing to be a sexual object).

✦ Attraction to "illicit" sexual activities such as pornography and prostitution.

✦ Anger and disgust at any public (or media) display of affection, sexuality, nudity, or partial nudity.

✦ Sexual manipulation, including using seductiveness or other forms of sexual manipulation to get what is wanted in martial, social, or business relationships; sexualizing all relationships (which can cause victims to become sexual victimizers of their own or other people's children).

✦ Sexual addiction, wherein victims, sexualized early on, often become addicted to daily sex or masturbation as a way of alleviating anxiety and comforting themselves.

As you can see, the experience of being sexually abused can have a tremendous effect on your child's ability to have healthy sexual relationships as an adult. For this reason it is essential that you make certain your child receives either individual or group psychotherapy. If your child was molested by someone in the family, the entire family will need professional help. Most communities have a community counseling center or mental healthy agency that provides low-cost counseling for sex abuse survivors and their families. The American Association of Sex Educators, Counselors, and Therapists (AASECT) can help you find a sex therapist in your area who specializes in working with children who have been sexually abused; their number is 312-644-0828.

IF YOUR TEEN IS RAPED

Many victims of rape feel tremendous guilt, blaming themselves for what happened. But this is the last thing you want your child to feel. She or he has enough healing to do without adding this unnecessary burden. Make certain that you don't in any way add to your child's feelings of guilt and shame by insinuating that the child was responsible in some way.

Whatever you may feel inside, this is not the time to blame your child. He or she needs reassurance and acknowledgment for having survived such an ordeal, not chastising with words like: "I warned you about wearing such sexy clothes," or "Maybe now you'll listen to me when I tell you to stay away from that crowd."

Even if you think you're right, don't say it. Your child needs to know that under no circumstances does she or he deserve such treatment. The rapist is always wrong, and the victim is always right.

What your child needs now is comfort and reassurance with statements like: "I'm so sorry this happened to you. I want you to know that I'll be here to support you in any way I can. Naturally, we have to make sure you're all right. We'll see that you get a medical checkup as soon as possible."

Your next task is to get your child to a hospital where there is a rape counselor available. There she or he can be medically checked for any injuries or possible STDs or pregnancy. Make sure your child doesn't change anything about her or his body—don't let the child take a bath or even comb her or his hair, and have the child leave her or his clothes as they are. Otherwise, she or he could destroy evidence.

Hospital officials can also gather evidence to use in court, should you and your daughter or son decide to prosecute. A trained rape counselor can be sensitive and helpful. A counselor can reinforce your efforts to reassure your daughter or son that she or he was in no way to blame.

The rape counselor can also help the family decide what to do about prosecuting the rapist. Talking to the police and giving evidence in court are difficult issues for most people, both old and young. Many report that they feel it is more humiliating to go through a court appearance than it is just to live with what happened. Teenage girls, in particular, often report that they can't stand the idea of going back to school and having classmates talk about it. They're sure that girls will tease them and that boys will cease to respect them. Often they're convinced that whatever popularity they had will vanish with disclosure.

It is important to let your child make the final decision about prosecuting. If you try to talk her or him into doing what you think is right, your child may get the message that she or he doesn't know what's best for her or himself. Since your child's self-esteem is already badly shaken, it is far more important to respect your child's opinion and abide by it. Providing that kind of reassurance is more important than any other kind of action you may take.

The last thing you want is for your child to begin seeing herself or himself as a victim because then she or he will start acting like one—afraid to assert her or himself, afraid to demand her or his rights.

If your daughter or son does decide to prosecute, you will need to encourage her or him to do so and be prepared to support her or him all the way. That means finding sympathetic lawyers, learning as much on the subject as possible, and staying in court with her or him.

There are other ways that your daughter or son will want your support, such as by not telling others, even other members of the family. If, for example, your daughter has only told you, her mother, you may feel that as a matter of principle, her father has the right to know what has happened. On the other hand, it may be better to respect your daughter's feelings and show her that you respect her decision. Share your preference with her, and then let her decide. Say, for instance: "I prefer that you tell your dad about it. I feel very uncomfortable keeping such a secret from him. But you're the one I'm most concerned about, and if you feel you can't tell him, I will respect your wishes. I do hope you will change your mind. You don't have to do it now. Just think about it."

If your daughter or son does decide to tell his or her father and/or siblings, their assurance and encouragement can be very beneficial. Comments like "You're my daughter (or son), and I love you more than ever," or "Hey, sis, you were really brave," can be a wonderful support. Don't be surprised, though, if she or he doesn't feel comfortable around males for a while and rebuffs their physical attempts to comfort her or him.

While you don't want your child to blame him or herself, you do want your child to feel her or his anger toward the rapist. Encourage your child to express this anger, by talking about it with you or a rape counselor, with physical forms of release such as shouting into a pillow or hitting the bed with a tennis racket, or by expressing it creatively through writing, art, or movement. The best thing for your child is to convert his or her shame to anger.

Of course, it's also natural for you to feel anger toward the rapist. By all means, share that with your child. In this way you can model ways for your child to release her or his anger.

WHAT TO EXPECT AS TIME GOES ON

Carrie's first experience with sexual intercourse was when she was date-raped at seventeen.

I was on my second date with a really popular guy at school, a football star. He was really nice to me the first part of our date, but later in the evening when we parked up on the hill where all the kids go to make out, he became really persistent. I tried to push his hands away gently, but he wouldn't take no for an answer. I started to become frightened and insisted that he take me home, but he just became more and more aggressive with me. Before I knew it, he had me pinned down on the front seat of the car and was forcing himself into me. I tried to scream for help, but he had parked so far away from the other cars that no one heard me.

Although it seemed like it took forever because the pain was so excruciating, it was all over within minutes and he was starting up the car. We drove home in silence, and he unceremoniously dropped me off in front of my house.

I know now that I should have told my parents and the authorities because God knows how many other girls he raped, but I was too ashamed. I felt responsible somehow, probably because he had called me a prick-tease while he was raping me. I was a virgin when he raped me, and I was more concerned about having lost my virginity and possibly being pregnant than I was about his being punished or even being stopped.

Needless to say, this experience was tremendously traumatic for Carrie. And as is true in many date rapes, Carrie didn't define what had happened to her as rape. Instead she blamed herself for parking with the boy in the first place and believed that she had indeed "led him on."

After this experience occurred, I felt a whole lot of shame. I imagined that everyone at school knew about it. I became extremely withdrawn and dropped out of most of the extra-curricular activities I had been involved in. Since I had gotten in trouble for being a 'prick-tease,' I started dressing much more conservatively and hardly looked at boys at all.

The trauma caused by Carrie's experience is typical of most women who are date-raped. Most experience a tremendous amount of shame, and most blame themselves for the rape.

Because they knew the rapist, most victims do not report the crime, and in fact, many do not even consider it a crime. Although they try to minimize it, the effects of date or acquaintance rape are often extremely severe, especially in cases like Carrie's when the rape was their first sexual experience.

In addition to feelings of shame, victims suffer from a myriad of symptoms, many of which are similar to those suffered by victims of child sexual abuse—difficulty trusting others, sleep disturbances, anxiety and panic attacks, fear of the dark, fear of being alone with a man, inability to have sex, feeling like used property, intense anger toward men, and self-hatred.

Boys and girls who have been raped have to suffer not only from the physical and emotional damage of the rape itself, but from the shame and humiliation so often connected with the crime. Many, like Carrie, end up feeling tainted and spoiled and fear that no one will ever want them sexually again. Others are so traumatized that they fear they will never again enjoy a sexual relationship.

Almost all victims of violence experience nightmares and flashbacks in which they relive the rape scene. Although people are distressed with the nightmares and flashbacks, it's normal to experience them, and it's all part of the healing process. It's nature's way of helping us heal, by reliving the terror until we can tolerate it and make peace with it. They may continue for weeks or even months. If your daughter or son complains about these phenomena, reassure her or him that they're normal and that it is actually good she or he is experiencing these symptoms because they are a sign of improving health.

She or he may also be more nervous and jumpy than usual. That, too, is a natural reaction to a stressful event.

Another common reaction is for your child to be afraid to date again. By all means, don't push her or him into dating, thinking it will make the child forget the whole episode faster. Respect her or his time schedule for healing. There is no set time for anyone to regain confidence. All too often people are encouraged to "get on with their lives" before they are ready or able to do so.

If, however, you feel your daughter or son isn't getting any better, you should definitely encourage her or him to go into therapy. If she or he can get into a group for young people who have also been raped, progress will be much faster. Your child will find out that she or he is not alone with what she or he feels and that others have survived this trauma. With the support of an understanding family and good friends, and therapy if needed, your child can successfully rebuild her or his life.

You may find yourself overwhelmed with rage as well as feelings of guilt and shame. Although there's no logical reason for you to feel guilty, you may nevertheless. You may be bombarded with a torrent of "If onlys": "If only I hadn't let her go out," "If only I'd said no," and so on. It can be helpful to work out some of this anguish with a sensitive, experienced person. You may need your own reassurance during this time, as well as a safe place to blow off steam. I recommend you consult a counselor, at least during the crisis. The rape counselor may be able to recommend someone.

Just because your child was a victim once doesn't mean she or he need ever be again. Nothing is more powerful than a survivor who is determined never to be victimized again.

8

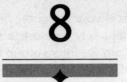

Teaching Sexual Values and Responsibility

Much has been said recently about the absence of values in our society and particularly about our failure to teach proper values to our children. We all agree that our children are in desperate need of values and guidance, but especially regarding their sexual behavior.

IS IT REALLY SO DIFFERENT FOR KIDS TODAY?

The answer is a resounding "YES." AIDS is certainly the most significant difference. Another is the fact that there is more *opportunity* for kids to have sex. While it is true that kids who want to have sex have always found a place to do it, the fact is that with single-parent families and two-parent working families, kids have more private access to their own homes. In a survey conducted by NBC News, 75 percent of kids who were having sex said they had it at their home or their partner's home.

And, there are other differences. The threat of AIDS notwithstanding, the stigma of having sex before marriage is blatantly absent. Even teenage girls who get pregnant are not ostracized by their classmates the way they once were. In fact, pregnant teens are envied and even admired in some social circles. Some pregnant teens admit to getting pregnant deliberately, either because they see it as a way of holding on to their boyfriend, because they "love" their boyfriend so much they think it is a way of having a part of him forever, or, as some teens report, because they want someone to love.

How do you raise a male child to become an adult who is capable of intimacy, sensuality, and commitment when his friends are talking about seeing how many girls they can "score" with, how many points they have, or how many girls they have in their "stable"? Conversely, how do you raise a girl to have self-respect and self-confidence when she constantly hears females referred to as whores and when the only way she can get a boy to pay attention to her is to have sex with him? The answer is by teaching your child *healthy sexual values*.

WHY TEACH VALUES?

Why teach values? Because teaching values is one of the most significant and effective things you can do for your child's long-term happiness. Values are the fundamental tools your child needs to face life's challenges.

Children need to be taught the moral aspect of sex as well as the physical and emotional aspects. While we can't mandate morals, those children who are raised from an early age to adhere to certain values concerning sex and their bodies are definitely going to have more respect for themselves and their bodies than those who are not.

With or without your help, your child will begin developing both conscious and unconscious values during his or her preschool years. Your child is like a sponge, taking in all that he or she sees and hears. He or she will begin to learn values from observing and interacting with friends and from watching television, but mostly he or she will learn them from listening to, observing, and interacting with the family.

If you avoid formally educating your child regarding values, he or she will receive the message from you that values aren't important. The value-developing process works best when parents consciously teach and set examples all along the way. Your child will still develop his or her own value system—but will do so because you showed that it was an important part of the child's development. Your child will test and develop and sometimes alter these values as he or she enters school. As your child approaches adolescence, he or she will struggle for autonomy and begin to set up his or her own value system that is independent of (but not usually different from) that of his or her parents.

"Should parents be the ones to teach values? Isn't that the job of the church?" you might ask. While the church is certainly a place for children to learn morals and values, sexual values are not discussed very often in churches today, and those that are tend to be rather narrow and rigid. (Later in this chapter, we will discuss how being rigid about values can backfire on you). In addition, many families do not attend church.

The two most important reasons why parents should be the ones to teach their child about sex and sexual morality are: 1) Parents can teach in a warm and loving way that avoids the sterile, factual, academic tone that predominates in school discussions; the silly or "dirty" connotation that often accompanies peer discussions; and the rigid and narrow tone of religious discussions. 2) When a parent teaches a child about sexual values, the intimate and personal nature of the subject creates a mutual sharing of trust and forms an emotional bond between parent and child.

There are basically two ways of learning: by trial and error and by gaining the wisdom of others. Certainly your child can learn all he or she needs to know about sexuality by going out and experiencing it, and he or she can learn all the lessons about fidelity, self-discipline, and so on, by making mistakes.

The failure and unhappiness of unhealthy behavior could cause your child to change. But learning morality and developing values through the school of hard knocks is a painful way to go. And one person's lifetime is not long enough to "invent the wheel"—to sort out all the connections between values and happiness. Therefore, passing along what you have already learned, teaching your child both the values and the connections, is a wonderful gift you can give him or her. It is no coincidence that the sages and seers of different cultures and countries have often taught the same basic values. That is because they have all learned through the centuries that certain values produce happiness and fulfillment.

PARENTS' DILEMMA: WHAT VALUES SHOULD I TEACH?

So what values should you teach your child? Before I tackle that one I'd better define the term *value*. Linda and Richard Eyre, in their book *Teaching Your Children Values* (see Bibliography and Recommended Reading), define values in this way:

> By *values* I mean the standards of our actions and the attitudes of our hearts and minds that shape who we are, how we live, and how we treat other people. Good values, of course, shape better people, better lives, and better treatment of others. . . . A true and universally acceptable value is one that produces behavior that is beneficial both to the practitioner and to those on whom it is practiced. It is a principle that either accomplishes well-being or prevents harm (or does both). It is something that helps or something that prevents hurt.

Parents today are caught up in a dilemma when it comes to deciding which sexual values to teach their children. First of all, those who grew up during the sexual revolution are confused because they want to provide their children with some of the freedom they enjoyed, but at the same time they are fearful because this kind of freedom will expose their children to AIDS and other sexually transmitted diseases. Parents who had originally intended to encourage their children to have full sex lives and not restrict them the way they were as children are now forced to warn their children of the dangers of AIDS and STDs.

Those more conservative parents who want to instill in their children certain religious values concerning sex are afraid to be too heavy-handed for fear of their children's rebelling—perhaps the way they themselves did as teenagers.

And parents who were sexually abused as children or raped as adults are afraid that their experiences will negatively affect their children, or that their fears might cause their children to become either overly fearful or the reverse, to become reckless.

Even those parents who consider themselves liberated and well-educated about sexuality sometimes feel hopelessly lost when it comes to what is going on with kids today.

No matter what their religious beliefs, most parents do not want to instill in their children the attitude that sex is a bad thing. Instead they want their children to grow up to be wise and honorable, to respect others, to be able to make good decisions, as well as to have a healthy sexual life. Unfortunately, although we live in the twentieth century, the archaic belief that sex is evil and dirty still lurks in our minds.

SOME IMPORTANT SEXUAL VALUES

Respect

We've lost something very precious in this society. In the past, young boys were raised to respect females, to treat them the way they would their mothers or sisters. This system left some things to be desired, of course. The madonna/whore syndrome was a lot more predominant. Males seldom married the girls they had sex with, but instead married the "good girls," the virgins.

But today, boys don't seem to respect *any* girl—the ones who "put out," or the ones who do not. In fact, many now seem to see it as a tremendous challenge to deflower virgins, exploit very young girls, and to manipulate those girls who resolve to remain chaste. We all remember the boys in Southern California who formed a club to see who could "score" the most points—one point for every girl they had sex with. Girls were just a number to them, nothing more. One girl was only twelve years old.

Many girls seem to be so desperate for a boyfriend that they will do anything to keep him—put up with his being unfaithful, risk AIDS, or have one or more babies with him outside of marriage. They don't respect themselves, and they don't seem to care (or perhaps they have just given up) whether the boy respects them or not.

Males should be taught that *all* girls are to be respected, no matter how they may be acting. Explain to your son that girls who act "cheap" and "easy" are often that way because they were sexually abused as a child, because they have low self-esteem, or because they are trying desperately to gain acceptance.

Teach your son to respect a girl's right to say "no." Teach him to respect his and the girl's body enough to wear a condom each and every time he has sex.

Females need to be taught that it is not worth gaining acceptance from others if in the process you disrespect yourself, and that a male who is able to manipulate or coerce a female into having sex is not a person who respects you. Female children need to be taught to demand respect from males and to respect themselves enough not to allow themselves to be used or abused by males. They also need to be taught to respect their bodies by insisting on using a condom if they do choose to have sex.

Honesty

Beginning when your child is nine or ten, you can have discussions about why people have sex. Watch for an opportunity (a

TV show or a video) to point out that there are basically six reasons for a male and female to have sex together:

1. Experimentation—a person does it to try out sex, to see how it feels.
2. Self-gratification—a person does it because he or she wants pleasure for him or herself.
3. Ego—a person does it to prove that he or she can.
4. Acceptance—a person does it to "be like everyone else" or to keep the other person from dropping or rejecting him or her.
5. Love—a person does it because he or she loves the other person and wants to give pleasure.
6. Love and commitment—a person does it because it is a way of showing not only love but commitment and trust and tenderness to his or her partner.

Point out that many teens have sex because of reasons 1 to 4. Depending upon your own values, you can teach your son that while it is understandable that he may want to have sex with a girl for reasons 1 and 2, it is dishonest for him to tell a girl he loves her in order to have sex. And having sex with a girl just to prove he can do it (because someone dared him, for example) is more than dishonest, it is abusive.

Girls need to be taught that boys will often tell them they "love" them in order to persuade them to have sex, but that generally they want to have sex for reasons 1 to 4. Explain that they may also be tempted to have sex for reason 4 (to gain acceptance), but that if a boy doesn't accept you the way you are, he won't accept you no matter what you do.

You may also want to point out that reasons 1 to 4 are not good reasons for having sex as a teenager because you run the risk of *hurting others or yourself.* When something as intimate as sex is done for reasons 1 to 4, it almost always leaves at least one of the parties feeling guilty, used, or selfish. If pregnancy occurs or a disease is contracted, the physical and emotional hurts get deeper and more complex. Even reason 5 can be a source of hurt (sometimes the most painful hurt) for adolescents because there is no commitment. For example, if a girl has sex with a boy just because she loves him, she risks being devastated if the relationship ends, or if she discovers he is unfaithful.

You may want to explain that when two people are in love, sex is a natural outgrowth of that love, a most intimate way of connecting with your loved one, and therefore reasons 5 and 6 are both good reasons to have sex. Reason 6 is seen by many to be the ultimate reason for having sex because it is more likely to provide both partners a certain level of security. However, most parents would be happy if their child's first sexual experience was with someone he or she loves because we all know that sex is more emotionally fulfilling when it is between people who love one another.

Fidelity and Chastity

Today, because of the constant threat of AIDS, it is easier than it has been for many decades to agree as a society on the desirability of abstinence before marriage and fidelity in marriage. Many parents who did not practice chastity or abstinence in their own youth are nonetheless hopeful that their children will. This is not hypocrisy. The fact that some of us have learned from our mistakes ought to be the best reason why our kids do not have to do likewise.

The value of remaining faithful to one person seems to have lost much of its significance for many males and even some females. Young males routinely have sex with several girls, all the while lying to each that she is the only one. Sadly, when the girl finds out that her boyfriend is sleeping around, she often puts up with it just to keep him.

The best time to teach your children the emotional benefits of fidelity within marriage is when they are very young. The underlying philosophy involved in teaching children the value of fidelity and chastity is that sex is too beautiful and too good to be given or used or thought of loosely or without commitment. It is natural for children to understand that after two people are married, sex is a bond and a special, private way of expressing love between them that should not be used outside marriage.

Help your child see the importance you place on this value as well as the happiness and security it gives you. Talk about commitment in personal terms, making your own example of fidelity as obvious and noticeable as possible. If you are a two-parent family, point out how the two of you belong to each other so that you don't need any other man or woman. Try to let your child see the basic physical signs of love and commitment, such as holding hands or kissing as you leave for work.

This is also a time to talk about AIDS and the danger of misusing sex. Describe who is helped by being careful about sex and who is hurt when people are not careful about it.

Unselfishness and Sensitivity

Females in our society tend to be more sensitive and unselfish than males in their dealings with other people. In fact, some people believe that females are socialized to be caretakers and nurturers and not to be selfish *enough* when it comes to their own needs. Males, on the other hand, tend to be more selfish in terms of wanting their own sexual needs to be met, sometimes to the detriment of a relationship. Females need to be taught to ask for what they want and to understand that they have a right to sexual pleasure. Males need to learn that a sensitive lover doesn't just think of his own needs and desires, but finds out what pleases his partner. Both sexes need to be taught that an important part of a loving relationship is to have a balance between making sure that your own needs are met and putting your own needs aside at times in order to please your partner.

Whatever your personal values are in terms of male and female roles, both male and female children need to be raised to have empathy for and be considerate of the feelings of the opposite sex. Girls need to be taught to be sensitive to the fact that boys get sexually aroused easier than they do. Males need to be taught that a good lover is one who is sensitive to the needs of his partner, who is tender, loving, and caring. If you teach your son to be macho and aggressive and that males are the dominant sex, don't be surprised if he also gets the message that it is okay to put his hands all over girls even if they don't want it and that it is okay to talk to girls in derogatory or overtly sexual ways. I will discuss this issue further in Part II.

Self-Control and Moderation

Both sexes need to be taught self-control and moderation. This includes alcohol and drug use as well as sexuality. As with most issues we have discussed, your child will learn the most about self-control and moderation from observing his or her parents' behavior. If you overindulge in food, alcohol, television, gambling, or any other substance, behavior, or activity, your child will probably not grow up to value self-control or moderation, but will follow in your footsteps.

Boys must be taught that they do not have the right to sexually harass young girls, the right to force themselves on girls, or to degrade them verbally.

HOW DOES A PARENT TEACH VALUES?

Ironically, it isn't as important *what* values you teach your child as *how* you teach them. Good guidance needs to start early on, not after a child has already reached sexual maturity. Don't wait for your child to come to you with questions about sex. Children can have questions without really knowing how to verbalize them. Or they may need to get comfortable with the topic of sex before they can ask you about their concerns. If they see that you are comfortable talking about sex, because they hear you talking openly about it with your adult friends or because you can talk openly with them, they will soon feel it is okay to talk to you no matter what the sexual issue.

DISCUSS, DON'T LECTURE

You can also teach values by asking your child questions, getting him or her to open up regarding what *he* or *she* thinks about a situation. Then you can share how you feel about it. In this way you aren't just lecturing, and he or she will be more likely to think later on about what you've discussed.

If something comes up in the news that relates to sexuality, use it as a springboard for discussion. For example, ask, "What do you think about those boys in California who had a club where they got points for every girl they had sex with?" Or, "How do you feel hearing that so-and-so is gay?" (Wait for a response.) "Do you respect him/her less?" (Wait again.)

Each time another celebrity comes out with the announcement that she or he has AIDS, or each time it is made public that someone is homosexual, you have a chance to have a discussion with your child: "How do you feel about the fact that Greg Louganis has AIDS?" (Wait for a response.) "Does it scare you?" (Wait again.) "Does it make you angry?" (Wait again.) After your child has responded, then you can share your own feelings.

During or after watching a television program or movie, you might say, "I don't approve of how women are being depicted in this movie," and then explain why. Ask your child his or her opinion as well. Talk openly with your partner or friends in front of your child about sexual values and ethics.

DON'T BE TOO RIGID OR HEAVY-HANDED

While it is important to teach children values, be aware that if you are too rigid in your beliefs, you may be setting your child up to rebel against you. We all know the story of the preacher's daughter who rebels against her father's rigidity by becoming promiscuous. This has in fact occurred so many times that it has become a cliché.

Be careful not to alienate your child with your strong beliefs and values. What you teach your child about such issues as homosexuality, male and female roles, pregnancy, and abortion is obviously your business. But remember, whether you are aware of it or not, your child will be strongly influenced by what you believe, one way or another. You may not want your child to become homosexual and may teach him or her that homosexuals are sinners; but if your child begins to think that he or she is one, do you want your child to hate himself or herself? Do you really want your child to believe he or she is worthless and evil? Or do you want your child to be able to come and talk to you about it?

Heavy-handedness does not work when it comes to teaching morals and values—sexual or otherwise. Children learn best by example. You are your child's most important role model. The way you conduct yourself in the presence of the opposite sex will send the loudest and strongest message. Living your life the way you would like your child to live his or hers is the best way to teach your child the sexual values and morals you would like him or her to know.

You can also offer your child other good examples of people who live healthy sexual lives and compare them with those who you feel do not. Be careful not to generalize about groups, but point to individuals, saying, for instance, "Do you know how Magic Johnson got AIDS? He got it from being promiscuous—having sex with a lot of women. He regrets it now, not only because he could get sick and die from the disease, but because now he is married and has a child, and he could have given them AIDS. Now that he has someone he loves, he wishes he hadn't done all that running around with other women. If you have a lot of sex when you are young, especially unprotected sex, you not only risk getting AIDS yourself, but you risk passing it on to the woman or man you will eventually want to marry and possibly even to your children."

If you catch your child doing something that goes strongly against your value system, instead of chastising him or her, talk to the child calmly, explaining why you disapprove of his or her actions. For instance, if you overhear your son bragging about

how he is "going steady" with three different girls and none of
them knows about the others, it is better to say quietly, "How
would you feel if a girl did that to you?" than to fly off the
handle.

Discuss your values and beliefs with your children. Tell them
why you hold those values and beliefs and how you feel you
have carried them out and how they have worked for you. For
example: "The reason I believe this is because my own life
experience has shown me that the important people in my life
are the ones who have made a commitment to me."

Share with your child the times when it was difficult for you
to stick to your beliefs, as well as the times when you did man-
age to stick to them. And tell him or her about how you think
you managed to carry them out even though it was difficult.
Use your own good judgment with this, of course, depending
on the age of your child and other circumstances (such as how
your disclosure will affect the family).

Have conversations about values, rather than lectures.
Conversations are two-way, with room for the exchange of
ideas, feelings, and information. It is as important for teens to
hear themselves voice their opinions as it is to hear you voice
yours.

Sometimes, if your child's opinions seem to be the opposite
of what you are conveying, it is difficult not to get angry or
worried and attack his or her ideas. But remember that saying
anything that cuts off communication reduces the opportunity
for your child to do further thinking and talking. The testing
out of values and beliefs is a process. Counter-values and
counter-ideas are an important part of that.

If you firmly believe that sex should be performed only
within a marital context, you will certainly want to convey
that to your child. However, be aware that the influences of
the society are strong. We live in a society where this is not
the predominant view. That means that through family,
friends, and social messages, young people are likely to be exposed to values other than yours.

TEACHING SEXUAL RESPONSIBILITY

As important as teaching sexual values is teaching sexual *responsibility*. Unfortunately, in many cases this may involve teaching things that go against your own value system. For example, AIDS is a serious threat to all teenagers, heterosexual as well as homosexual, non-drug-users as well as those using a needle, white as well as black or Hispanic. Teaching your teen (female and male) *always* to use a condom if he or she is going to have sex may seem to you to be giving permission for the teen to have sex. But think of it this way: How would you feel if you found out your child did have sex and did *not* use a condom? If you have done your job teaching your child what you consider to be good values, then you must be willing to let go and trust that your teachings have worked as well as they are going to. We all know that it is difficult to always live up to what we believe in, to always act in the way we believe we should. Teens are no exception. In fact it is even more difficult for teens, with their raging hormones, to maintain control over their impulses. A good analogy to this would be the fact that you more than likely don't want your teen to drink and have probably made that very clear. On the other hand, you know that it is a common occurrence for teens to experiment with alcohol (as you probably did). Could you imagine yourself saying, "I don't want you to drink, but if you do, make sure you have a designated driver"? Does this sound to you like you are giving your child permission to drink, or that you are being realistic and teaching your child about responsible drinking?

Parents also need to carefully consider personal sexual values against the reality of changing, more liberal values of society. Nowadays, for example, teenagers will often have their first sexual experience at a time, an age, or in a way that the parent doesn't approve of. Although parents often find they cannot control their teenager's sexuality, there are numerous ways in which parents can at least influence their teenager's sexual activities.

For example, parents must help their teenager understand that engaging in intercourse requires a decision. The teen needs to understand that he or she should not engage in intercourse simply because he or she has an impulse to do so. Instead, the first sexual experience should come only after careful consideration.

Many parents suggest or insist that their child be in love before they become sexual. Love does make a first sexual experience more meaningful and pleasurable, but love should not be the only condition one should consider before becoming sexual. Many teenagers fall in and out of love as often as they change their clothes, while other teenagers fall madly and passionately in love with the wrong people.

I suggest that parents stress another, equally important criterion for a sexual relationship—and that is a feeling of trust with the other person. Teaching a teenager how to evaluate a person's trustworthiness is often difficult. Questions that help teenagers to evaluate trustworthiness include:

+ Is this person consistent in the way he or she treats me?
+ Does this person talk about people behind their backs?
+ Does this person divulge things told to him or her in confidence (secrets) with other people?
+ Is this person loyal?
+ What does this person say about his or her previous partners?

And today, in the age of AIDS, determining whether a potential sex partner is a safe physical risk is also important. While it should be stressed to teenagers that there is no foolproof way to protect themselves from AIDS short of celibacy, choosing partners carefully is certainly an important safeguard. Therefore, choosing a potential sex partner should also involve finding out:

+ Does this person *always* practice safe sex?
+ How much sexual experience has this person had?
+ What kind of partners has this person had?

✦ Is this person an intravenous drug-user?
✦ Is this person bisexual?

Children also need to be taught the consequences of having sex—what is going to happen to his or her life if he or she becomes pregnant, gets someone pregnant, or contracts a venereal disease.

If your child's school has a sex education program or is thinking of having one, get involved. *The Complete Guide to Safe Sex*, a book written by The Institute for Advanced Study of Human Sexuality, encourages you to do your best to insure that the curriculum is accurate, extensive, and value-balanced with the three Rs: Rights, Responsibilities, and Rewards of sexuality. The book states that everyone has the *Right* to sexual expression that is not exploitive of others. Everyone, in being sexual, assumes *Responsibility* for the results of one's sexual activity on oneself, one's partner, one's family, and society. Everyone can enjoy the *Rewards* of sexuality, which include physical pleasure, emotional closeness, spiritual union, procreation, relaxation, and physical and psychological health.

As a parent imparting sexual information to your teenager, you may function best as a consultant. A consultant is an expert who gives information, opinions, and/or recommendations without assuming responsibility for the ultimate decision. If the school provides the facts, you can discuss the feelings and balance out the impact with family values. Young teens, when faced with the complexities and consequences of adult sexual behavior, may declare that a life of celibacy is the best way to deal with it all. It is a perfect choice for the moment, and you may be tremendously relieved. But they need some indication from you that their resolve may weaken as their hormones kick into high gear and that there are joys and rewards that are unique to sexual sharing.

The government is spending over five million dollars on "chastity education" under the guise of AIDS prevention. While abstinence may seem to be a simple and effective solution, it is unrealistic to believe that the majority of young people will wait more than a decade after pubescence to explore their sexuality. Surveys on teenage sexuality and developmental psychology pinpoint mid-adolescence as the time of biological and psychological readiness to begin relationships that will lead to sexual sharing. Many youngsters who have the desire and the opportunity will experiment sexually on a more casual basis in their early teens. It is more reasonable for you to accept that your adolescent will be sexual at a time that he or she will choose and that you can be influential in this decision by respecting his or her maturation and preparing the adolescent for adult privileges and responsibilities.

According to *The Complete Guide to Safe Sex*, your most important task with the early teenager is to prepare your son or daughter to look forward to the rewards of sexual sharing despite our increasingly unhealthy sexual world. Although you can't scare him or her out of being sexual, you can certainly undermine the joys of sexual intimacy by instilling fear and guilt. Help your early teenager by endorsing sex as a legitimate area of concern, by acknowledging that sexual sharing is a healthy, pleasurable human experience, and by emphasizing that his or her sexual choices will have a significant impact (good and bad) on his or her own life and the lives of others and society at large.

Instead of "prohibiting" early sexual involvement, give your adolescent a clear understanding of the risks and responsibilities involved with sexual activity. Tell your child the reasons for the desirability for sexual abstinence prior to marriage:

+ Physical reasons—AIDS and other STDs, pregnancy.
+ Emotional reasons—the hurt and insecurity that can result.
+ Social reasons—the desirability of a respected rather than a "loose" reputation.
+ Mental reasons—interference with the ability to focus on academic and other mental pursuits.
+ Religious reasons—if these are important to you.

Explain why early sexual promiscuity occurs and provide a workable, practical formula for avoiding it. Tell your teen that studies have shown that most boys who become involved in teenage sex do it for *ego* reasons (to prove their manhood, to exploit someone, to show they can do it, to brag to their peers), whereas girls do so for *emotional* reasons (desire to be accepted or not rejected, for warmth, security). Ask your teen if either of these is a good reason.

Many teens (and preteens) have sex for reasons other than pure sexual interest. Some choose to have sex because they are lonely, some do it as a way of rebelling, some do it because of peer pressure ("Everyone else is doing it"), and some do it to be popular. Teaching your child about the good reasons to have sex (love and commitment) is an important part of his or her education.

AFTER VALUES, TRUST AND ACCEPTANCE

Finally, while you want to be able to instill in your children the proper values, you must learn to trust them enough and give them enough space to have their own experiences and develop their own set of values.

Let your children know that no matter what happens to them (venereal disease, pregnancy, abortion), they can come to you for help, even if they have done something against your values.

Say, for example, "I would never want you to feel that you couldn't come to me and tell me anything, even if you thought I wouldn't approve. Please know that I love you and that we could work out anything together. I might not approve of something you've done, but I will always love you and want to be there for you."

Whether you are Jewish, Catholic, Fundamentalist Christian, or Buddhist, whether you are conservative or liberal, a free spirit, a staunch feminist, a pro-lifer or a pro-choicer, in addition to teaching your children about your beliefs and values you will also need to:

✦ Follow your own rules and not be a hypocrite.
✦ Teach tolerance for others' differences.
✦ Teach your children to respect and honor their bodies and those of others.

In summary:

✦ Get clear about your own values (see "Parental Issues" at the end of the chapter).
✦ Get clear about what you want your child to learn about sex. What do you most want to teach your child about sex?
✦ Prepare the answers that you want to give if your child asks you a question.
✦ Don't wait until your child comes to you with questions; initiate talks about sexuality.
✦ Model your values: Be a good example of the kind of person you want your child to be and participate in the kind of relationship you want your child to have.
✦ Make sure your values are not so rigid that your child rejects them or feels he or she can't live up to them.
✦ Don't overwhelm your child with rules, especially rules she or he can't possibly live up to in today's world.
✦ Teach your child that no matter what, he or she can come to you.

PARENTAL ISSUE: WHAT ARE YOUR BELIEFS AND VALUES?

It is vitally important that you get in touch with your own ideas about sex, to become clear about your sexual beliefs and values so you will be better equipped to communicate them to your children in simple, direct terms. If you can put your ideas into words, you will have a better understanding of what those ideas are and be better able to teach them clearly and respond constructively to the curves your children are likely to pitch to you.

Behavior includes everyday acts like locking the bathroom

door. Beliefs include things like equality of the sexes, "double standards," or sexual fidelity.

For example, how do you feel about the difference between boys and girls? Do you feel that boys are more likely to engage in sex than girls? Do you consider girls "purer" than boys? Do you see boys as being able to take "purity" away from girls? Do you see girls as sexual victims and boys as sexual aggressors?

Now let's consider how you feel about men being "macho"—aggressive and dictatorial—or "manly," and how that relates to your style as a role model for your children. In your view, should males be macho or manly in their attitude toward sex and the performance of sex? Does that mean that men "lead" in sexual approaches and actions? Should a man initiate sex, direct it, and be in charge of the scenario? He might do that roughly or gently, but is he the one in charge? Should women expect that? Are you going to teach your daughter to expect it, put up with it, or resist it? Are you going to teach your son to take that stance?

Here are some more questions to ask yourself:

- ✦ Do you support women's rights?
- ✦ Do you believe in an equal relationship between males and females?
- ✦ Do you model this kind of relationship to your children?
- ✦ Do you believe that there should be a clear distinction in sex roles for women and men?
- ✦ Do you think girls should be feminine and frilly?
- ✦ Do you think females should ever invite or initiate sex?
- ✦ Do you believe in birth control?
- ✦ Do you feel females should be responsible for contraception?
- ✦ Are shy boys "safer" for girls to date?
- ✦ Are homely girls more likely to be "pushovers"?
- ✦ Do you have a lock on your bedroom door?
- ✦ Should children know if their parents make love?
- ✦ Do you believe in the "double standard"—that men can be promiscuous but women should not?

✦ Would you prefer your daughter to be a virgin when she marries?
✦ How about your son?
✦ Do you believe young people should get experience sexually before marriage and commitment?
✦ Would you prefer that your child live with someone before getting married?
✦ Do you believe that whatever two consenting adults do sexually is okay?
✦ What about two consenting adolescents?
✦ If you had it to do over, what would you change about your adolescent sexual behavior?
✦ Would you discuss that with your adolescent child?
✦ What are your views on abortion?
✦ What are your views on homosexuality?

These are just some of the questions you might want to ask yourself regarding your sexual beliefs and standards. They will help you to clarify your sexual attitudes. Knowing what your sexual attitudes are will help you to understand them and how they might influence your child.

By teaching your child your sexual values, you aren't limiting her or him, but rather giving your child the foundation from which to build her or his character and a frame of reference from which to begin to develop her or his own sexual values.

By teaching sexual responsibility, you are teaching your child to respect the rights of others and in so doing are making it more possible for your child to have his or her own rights respected.

And last, but certainly not least, teaching sexual values and responsibility will teach your child to value him or herself and others.

9

♦

Raising a Sensuous Child

Raising a sensuous child may or may not seem to be an important issue for you as a parent. But think about it for a moment. Sensuality is an important part of a good sexual relationship. It is what distinguishes a loving, intimate bonding between two people from pure animalistic sex. Touching, caressing, holding, and kissing are as important in lovemaking as the act of intercourse.

We all experience the importance of touch and sensuality in different ways. Those of you whose parents believed in the importance of touch, who gave you adequate nurturing and caressing, have known the pleasures of physical touch both as a receiver and a giver. You know the importance of sensuality in your life, the benefits and the opportunities it affords for expressing intimacy and love.

Those of you who were raised by parents who gave very little physical nurturing, who may even have deprived you of physical touch, know firsthand how such deprivation can affect a child's self-esteem and ability to become intimate. Those who were not touched, who were taught that touch was dangerous (such as those who were seemingly rejected by parents when they reached out, or those who were sexually abused), almost always grow up to be adults who are either afraid of touch and intimacy, or who are so shut-down that they cannot feel the pleasures of physical touch.

What is sensuality exactly? The dictionary defines *sensuous* as relating to or consisting of the gratification of the senses or the indulgence of appetite. Sensuality is at the very heart of our sexuality. Our ability to receive and appreciate the pleasure our senses give us is intimately linked to our ability to be fully sexual. A child who is encouraged to explore and value his or her senses will most certainly grow up to enjoy a loving, sexual relationship far more than one who is not.

WHY TEACH SENSUALITY?

In addition to helping us become intimate and enhancing our sexual relationships, sensuality should be taught to our children and teens as a viable alternative to sex. If we are going to teach our children to abstain from sex and make them aware of the dangers of STDs and AIDS, we need also to encourage them to explore their sensuality.

All through our lives we experience times when sexual intercourse is not possible (for example, during the latter months of pregnancy, or because of illness, vaginal infections in women, impotency in men, and the effects of aging). Because of this it is important that you teach your child that there are alternatives—sensual alternatives to intercourse and sex.

And finally, as discussed in Chapter Four, "Raising a Child with a Healthy Body Image," it is vitally important that you help your child stay connected to her or his body in order for the child to maintain a positive body image. There is no better way to do this than to encourage your child to explore her or his senses.

Teaching your child to be sensuous is really more about not robbing your child of his or her natural sensuality—not discouraging your child from being his or her sensuous self—than anything else. Children are naturally sensuous. In fact, children can teach adults a lot about noticing their environment—paying attention to colors, sounds, and other textures of life.

YOUR BABY'S FIRST BODY FEELINGS

The first pleasurable sensations a baby enjoys come through his or her mouth. Lips are particularly sensitive. Feeding not only satisfies hunger but satisfies the strong natural need to suck. It is through his or her lips that your baby makes his or her first warm contact with another human being, forms his or her first relationship, and finds his or her earliest love—Mother.

A baby who is allowed plenty of time to enjoy feeding and sucking at his or her own pace takes in love and food and warmth, while at the same time his or her tension, empty feeling, and discomfort subside. And unless a baby has some special physical discomfort, is especially tense, or falls asleep during feeding, he or she feels satisfied and is at peace with the world.

As soon as babies have learned to use their hands, they find out that it gives them pleasure to touch not only their mouths but also their thumbs, toes, and ears. A very young baby seems to use his or her thumb as a substitute for the nipple—a way of continuing the sucking he or she does at breast or bottle. By the time babies are six months or so, they may find that sucking the thumb brings comfort—at bedtime, or when they are tired or fearful or don't feel well. It may also remind them of early closeness with mother.

In addition, babies have their own special do-it-yourself comforters such as soft blankets, fuzzy toy animals, a wisp of hair to twirl, or anything they like to clutch or suck on. Babies turn to these to make up for life's inevitable letdowns or for any shortages in the sucking that is so important to them. These pacifiers, other than thumbs, are referred to by Dr. D. W. Winnicott, the British psychoanalyst and child psychiatrist, as "transitional objects." This grasping indicates that the baby has formed a kind of relationship to something—not as close as to the baby's mother or his or her thumb, but a relationship to an object that is outside of both. It also is a step in growing up, although it certainly doesn't look it. Babies will protest loudly and vehemently if deprived of their much-needed symbol of security.

Toward the end of the first year or so, as a baby gets to know more about his or her body, the baby may discover that touching his or her genital area also brings a pleasant sensation. It seems to be more soothing than stimulating. Sometimes a child will find his or her genitals just before going to sleep.

Needless to say, these pleasant explorations and transient touchings are quite harmless, and as stated earlier, it is wise not to discourage them. Babies soon become aware of the gestures and expressions on their parents' faces. A look of disapproval, the pulling away of the baby's hand, or a verbal "Mustn't touch" may only awaken or further stimulate the baby's interest in this section of his or her anatomy, or give the baby the idea that there is something "bad" about this part of their bodies. Usually, at this age, the baby's interest in his or her genitals is only a passing one, for the baby is now beginning to become absorbed by the exciting things in the world outside his or her body.

The surface of an infant's skin is extremely sensitive. It responds to the caressing water of the bath, to being stroked and fondled and soothed by the hands of those who care for him or her. These good body feelings help the baby form a healthy image of his or her own body. A baby soon begins to associate these pleasant sensations with Mother or Father or the caretaker who brings them to him or her, and they strengthen the baby's growing bond with that person.

There is no time aside from feeding time in which a parent and child can participate in more mutual delight than in the ritual of the daily bath. Most babies come to love the feel of the warm water touching their skin. One mother, describing her baby's reactions, stated, "He literally gurgles and snorts with joy as he pulls up his tiny legs and then kicks them out again." An infant sometimes squeals with pleasure as he or she is dried and patted with a soft towel and then feels the cozy sensations of a clean diaper and fresh clothes.

ENCOURAGING YOUR CHILD'S NATURAL SENSUALITY

Although children are born with the ability to appreciate their senses, all too often, young children have this appreciation forced away from them. Children need encouragement to continue their natural appreciation. Make sure that potentially sensuous activities like eating, bathing, and dressing are not turned into either routine, mundane chores or even dreaded events, as in the case of April.

When April was a little girl her mother was very serious about making sure her daughter was clean. She would run a tub of extremely hot water, tell April to get in it, and then scrub her so hard that it almost made her skin raw. Today, April refuses to take baths if there is a shower available. She showers quickly in almost-cold water. Her husband complains that they can never enjoy the luxurious sensuality of a relaxing bath together.

Parents often lose track of the fact that a bath can do more than just clean your child. If you rush your child in and out of the bathtub in the interest of time, you are robbing her or him of the experience of relaxing in the warm water, feeling the sensuousness of the water on his or her skin. Nothing relaxes a child (or an adult) more than a warm bath. The next time you find yourself rushing your child out of the bathtub, remember how good a bath feels. Better yet, remind yourself to take the time for a leisurely bath yourself.

Make meals an opportunity for sensuous enjoyment for your child. Allow her or him plenty of time to explore her or his senses instead of rushing through the task. It is far more important for children to learn to enjoy the different textures of food than it is for them to finish their meal quickly. (Notice how toddlers who are newly introduced to food spend more time playing with it than eating it. This is a natural developmental process.) You can help develop your children's natural sensuality by allowing them to play in the mud or snow, spending extra time in the bath, or teaching them the joys of preparing and eating different flavors and textures of food. Call their attention to sensory information, such as asking them to describe a certain taste, smell, texture, sound, or sight. For instance: "How does this food taste?" or "What is the most beautiful thing you saw on our walk?" or "Do you feel the wind on your face?" This will teach children to attend to their senses. Here are some other suggestions:

- ✦ If you have a dog or cat, point out how soft its fur is, how its fur has different textures in various parts of its body.
- ✦ Take the petals off a rose. Let your child feel the softness against his or her skin, on his or her lips.
- ✦ Listen to a variety of different kinds of music with your child, and, if he or she seems to enjoy dancing, encourage it.
- ✦ Ask your child how he or she imagines it might feel to lie down on clouds, to sleep on rose petals, to roll around on the green grass.

THE JOYS OF SENSUAL TOUCH

One of the best ways for you to encourage your child's natural sensuality is for you to introduce her or him to the joys of sensual touch. This will begin when your child is still an infant, when you caress and soothe her or his skin softly with your fingertips, when you apply oil or powder tenderly, when you softly smooth your child's brow, arms, legs, and feet, and when you bathe her or him gently with soapsuds. All through his or her childhood, you can show your child that touching can be comforting, nurturing, and stimulating.

Although there will come a time when your child will bathe herself or himself (at approximately five years old), you can encourage your child to continue leisurely baths by not rushing her or him and by telling the child that you know how good the warm water feels on his or her skin.

And while you will not need to continue towel-drying your child after the age of five, you can provide a large, soft towel for the child to dry herself or himself gently the way you once so lovingly did.

Most important, you will need to continue physical contact with your child throughout the school-age years. Continue to demonstrate your affection through hugs, kisses, and pats on the shoulder. And you can continue to caress your child throughout his or her life, soothing the child's brow when he or she is ill, gently rubbing his or her back to lull the child to sleep, lovingly stroking his or her arms as your child sits beside you.

If you were seldom touched as a child, you know the limitation it has imposed on you. Don't pass this legacy on to your child.

You have taught your daughter or son about good touch/bad touch, and your intentions are good, so there is no reason to stop touching your child just because he or she is getting older. As long as your child asks for the touch, or genuinely seems to like it (you can tell by whether he or she stiffens or shrinks from your touch, or relaxes into the touching), and as long as you are not attempting to satisfy your own unmet needs and are not feeling sexual or attempting to sexually stimulate your child, there is no reason why you shouldn't continue to touch her or him appropriately all during childhood. In so doing you will be teaching her or him that touch is an important part of intimacy.

It is important, however, that you not ask for nor allow your child to caress or massage you. (Simply stroking your hand or arm or foot is, of course, perfectly acceptable.) What is not acceptable is for you to ask your child to massage your back, buttocks, thighs, or stomach.

If you were sexually abused as a child, you may be afraid to touch your child for fear of losing control or of giving your child the wrong idea. But neither do you want to raise a child who is deprived of touch, who doesn't know that touch is an important avenue for showing love and concern. If you actually feel aroused when touching your child (other than while breast-feeding, as discussed earlier), then by all means do not continue. But if you do not experience such feelings, it is safe to say that touching your child will only do good for her or him and for you.

MODELING SENSUALITY

The best form of sensuality training, of course, is parental modeling. As mentioned earlier, children need to see their parents being affectionate with one another. And they need to see their parents enjoying other sensuous pursuits such as stopping to smell the roses and appreciating art and music.

In addition, comment as often as possible on how different things—such as the scenery, the weather, food, fabrics, and so on—affect you: "Isn't that a beautiful sunset? Look at all the colors," or "I love it when it rains and makes everything smell so fresh and clean," or "Isn't this soup good? I love a soup that is thick and creamy like this."

Certain sports and activities, such as gymnastics, swimming, running, and dancing, encourage sensuality because they foster an appreciation of one's body. In addition, children's sensuality can be encouraged by teaching an appreciation of art and music.

I have offered many suggestions in this chapter, some of which may sound strange to you, some of which will be uncomfortable for you to do. The important thing is that you encourage your child to hold on to his or her natural sensuality and that you give your child permission to explore all his or her senses. You can do this in whatever ways are comfortable and natural for you. If you are an artist, you may do it by encouraging your child to experiment with clay or finger paints. If you are an athlete, you will do it by teaching your child to appreciate his or her body. If you are a nature buff, it will be through the appreciation of nature.

CONTINUE YOUR TRAINING INTO YOUR CHILD'S ADOLESCENCE

When your child is an adolescent, teach her or him that there are many ways other than sexual activity to have intimate contact. In fact, sexual contact is only one possibility of sensual touch. There is a continuum of sensual touch, progressing from less sexual to more sexual kinds of touch. This continuum begins with holding, hugging, and kissing, and moves up to stroking, massage, and sexual pleasuring.

Explain to your adolescent that our entire body, from the top of our heads to the soles of our feet, is a virtual banquet of potential sensual and erotic delights. If your teen doesn't feel ready for any kind of sexual activity, encourage her or him to find acceptable alternatives and to work with his or her partner to develop mutually pleasurable, nonsexual touch experiences such as massage and cuddling. Neither the limitations created by your adolescent's value and belief systems, his or her determination to remain a virgin until marriage, or the threat of AIDS need diminish the abundance of sensual experiences available to her or him.

Encourage your teen who is ready for sexual activity to view safe sex as an opportunity to explore and play, to be truly spontaneous. When this occurs, it becomes an adventure— one that continues to bring new zest and thrill to our love lives.

Explain to your teen that too often we focus all our attention on our genitals when making love. There are other parts of the body that can be just as erotic and feel just as pleasurable when touched. Men in particular tend to focus all their attention on the penis and on ejaculation as opposed to intimacy and pleasure. As a result of exploring a variety of ways of expressing intimacy, your teen will become far less compulsive and goal-oriented when it comes to sex. Exploring our personal sexual feelings, desires, sensuality, and eroticism is both a gift to ourselves and to those we love.

To summarize, sensuality training will help your child to:

+ Maintain his or her natural sensuality
+ Help him or her to have more fulfilling, intimate love relationships
+ Help him or her to stay connected to his or her body
+ Help him or her to postpone sex by offering other outlets for his or her sexual energy and intense feelings for another person
+ Teach him or her alternatives to intercourse in the age of AIDS and other STDs
+ Offer him or her a viable alternative to use in place of intercourse throughout his or her life

PARENTAL ISSUE: RECONNECTING WITH YOUR OWN SENSUALITY

One of the great things about being a parent is that you can learn right along with your child. All the suggestions that I made for you to encourage your child's natural sensuality (taking leisurely baths, taking the time to notice textures and tastes) will help you to reconnect with your own sensuous feelings. This in turn will help you be more inclined to model this kind of behavior for your children.

◆

EXERCISE

Collect a variety of objects that you find pleasurable to touch, smell, taste, listen to, or look at. Put your objects in a basket, bowl, or special box. Your sensory basket might include such things as satin cloth, polished rocks, feathers, flower petals, fruit, bells, and jewelry.

Spend a few minutes focusing on each object. Hold each

object, feel its texture, smell it, taste it, or listen to it. Decide which are your favorites. Have fun, experiment. Now share your basket with your child.

◆

THE IMPORTANCE OF TOUCH

Many of us have grown so accustomed to getting all our needs for intimacy met through sexual activity that we are unable to feel and express intimacy any other way. For many people, sex is the only way they really feel loved, yet there are many other ways of sharing intimacy, many ways of expressing love for one another besides being sexual: holding hands, caressing and massaging, taking a bath or Jacuzzi together, cuddling, scratching each other's back, or just taking a walk together.

In addition, many people view foreplay strictly as a preliminary activity, a kind of appetizer, with intercourse being the main course. But it doesn't have to be that way. Many couples enjoy satisfying sexual activity (including orgasm) that consists only of "foreplay activities," such as stimulation of the genitals by hand, tongue, or mouth. This shouldn't be seen as any less "vital" than intercourse, and it can be just as satisfying for both partners.

We live in a highly sexual culture that is not very sensual (body contact that is pleasurable but not erotic). Our entire culture tends to focus on genital sex and disregards the pleasures of other kinds of physical contact. Even lovers don't seem to touch as much as they want. Although this is usually not true in the beginning of a relationship, it is almost inevitable that once a relationship becomes sexual, the nonsexual touching declines sharply.

Touching is important to us our entire lives, so much so in fact that the amount and quality of our nonsexual touching experiences are intimately related to how satisfied we are with our sexual activities. "Why is this?" you might ask, "Just what does touching have to do with the quality of my sexual behavior?" The answer is that for most people, their sexual experiences are best, and the chances for avoiding sexual problems are highest, when they have sex only when it is sex that they want. When you use sex in an attempt to satisfy nonsexual needs such as the need for comforting, the need for reassurance, or the need for physical contact, you run the risk of becoming disappointed. Sex that is motivated by other needs is often unsatisfying and can even lead to sexual problems since our bodies usually respond to what we *really want*. If all you really want is a hug, your body may refuse to respond sexually to even the most erotic touches.

When you only share physical contact and affection in the context of sexual activity, sex takes on an exaggerated importance. Sex becomes weighed down with all the needs that aren't being met elsewhere. Ask yourself what you really want when you think you want sex. Is it closeness to someone you care about, a feeling of connectedness? Is it understanding or support? Is it reassurance that the person you care about cares about you in return? Or is it intercourse or orgasm?

Once you have some idea of what you want at any given time, ask yourself what the best way of getting it might be. Do you really just need a hug or to be held? Or do you need to connect with your partner by having an intimate conversation, perhaps including the request for some verbal reassurance? How would giving or receiving a massage feel? If you begin to take the time to ask yourself these questions, you will find that you will also begin to get your sexual needs and desires fulfilled in sex and satisfy needs for other kinds of contact and affection in more appropriate ways.

There will, of course, be times when sex is exactly what you want and need. But consider the following exercises for those times when sensual touch is more appropriate for your needs and desires.

SENSATE FOCUS EXERCISES

The following exercises are called "sensate focus" exercises and originated with the work of the sex therapists Masters and

Johnson. In my practice, they have helped hundreds of couples suffering from a vast variety of sexual and intimacy problems. They are designed to help establish trust between the couple and to help the couple find alternative ways of touching and sharing intimacy. The term "sensate focus" refers to the fact that during the exercises you are to *focus* your attention as closely as you can on your *sensations*, how it *feels* to touch or be touched. For example, whether you are the one who is giving the touch or receiving it, make sure that you always focus all your attention on the point where your body comes in contact with your partner's skin. If your mind wanders off during the exercise, bring it back to the exact point between your skin and your partner's skin.

This way of touching, called caressing, has been proven to remove the pressure to perform, to allow each person to touch for his or her own pleasure, and to help express tenderness, caring, and gentleness.

Caressing is different from massage or even what is commonly called "sensual massage," because instead of manipulating the large muscles of the body, you will be focused on the skin. Caressing is a slow, sensuous touch that is much lighter than massage and is done very, very slowly, using not just the tips of your fingers but your entire hand and even your forearm. Using the flat of your hand, you will caress your partner's skin with long sweeping strokes using the flat of your fingers, your palm, wrist, and forearm.

Another difference between caressing and massaging is that massage is intended solely for the pleasure or therapeutic benefit of the person *receiving* the massage, while caressing is done for the pleasure of the person *giving* the caress as well. You may have noticed in the past that you became tired easily while giving a massage and may even have become anxious because you were so concerned as to whether you were doing it *right* and pleasing the person you were giving the massage to. While the person receiving the caress certainly does enjoy it, the person giving the caress enjoys it equally, and since you are not worried about how well you are performing, it will not feel like a task but a pleasure.

To understand exactly what I mean, try the following:

Imagine that your right hand is the "giver" and your left hand is the "receiver." Touch your left hand using only the fingertips of your right hand. Which of your hands feels the pleasure of the touch? Most people will say that their left hand, the "receiver," feels the pleasure. But what about your right hand, does that hand feel any pleasure? Most people say "no," they don't feel any pleasure by using their fingertips.

Now try giving to the left hand by using the flat of your right hand, wrist, and the flat of your fingers. Which hand feels the pleasure of the touch this time? Most people will say that *both* hands feel pleasure, both the "giver" and the "receiver." Indeed, it is hard to tell which hand is the "giver" and which is the "receiver" when you use the caress technique.

The next exercise will help to build trust and provide each person with a feeling of being loved and wanted for reasons other than sexual ones.

---------------- ◆ ----------------

THE FOOT CARESS

You may do this exercise one of two ways, either including a foot bath or not. If you leave out the bath, all you need is some oil or lotion and two towels. If you would like to include the foot bath, you will need two towels, a basin or tub large enough for a person's feet, liquid soap, lotion, and hot water.

The foot bath can be a loving, relaxing part of this exercise and should be included if at all possible. The foot bath also solves the problem of having to worry about whether or not your feet smell or are sweaty.

---------------- ◆ ----------------

When You Are the Active Partner

Fill the basin with warm water and place your partner's feet in the water. If you do not have a basin large enough for both feet, do one foot at a time. Add the liquid soap and slowly caress your partner's feet in the water. Remember to touch for your own pleasure, using a light touch, not a massage. Bathe one foot at a time, finding out how the different areas of the foot feel as you bathe them. Spend at least five minutes on each foot, but you can take longer if you like.

When you are finished with both feet, lift each foot out of the water firmly but gently, dry them, and wrap them in separate towels. Put aside the basin. Now gently take one foot from the towel and caress it using the oil or lotion. Take as long as you like, staying longer on parts of the foot, ankle, and lower calf that you especially enjoy touching. Spend at least five to ten minutes on each foot.

Always maintain contact with your partner as you are giving the caress to avoid surprising her or him with a sudden touch when you switch hands. If you use lotion or oil, warm it in your hand before you apply it, and maintain contact with your partner's body when you reapply the lotion.

Make sure that you are going very, very slowly—the slower the better. If you think you are moving your hand slowly enough, cut your speed in half and see how this affects your ability to focus on the touch. Do not worry about whether your partner is enjoying the caress. It will be his or her responsibility to let you know if you are doing something uncomfortable.

While it is normal to become distracted now and then, if you find your mind wandering, try bringing it back to the place where your skin makes contact with your partner's skin.

Do not speak while doing the exercise, and do not ask for feedback during the exercise. Assume that the caress feels good or at least neutral.

When You Are the Passive Partner

To start, the passive person sits in a chair with his or her feet on the floor. Since this exercise includes the ankles and part of the calves, you will need to have your pant legs rolled up or wear shorts.

As the passive person during the foot bath and caress, all you need do is relax, enjoy, and allow yourself to be pampered. If your partner does something that bothers you, say something, but otherwise concentrate totally on the touch. Relax your feet and just let them hang from your legs. Your partner will lift them into the basin and move them—you don't need to help.

Close your eyes and try to relax any muscles that feel tense. Keep your attention on the place where your partner is touching your skin. Mentally follow your partner's hand as it caresses your body. Do not give your partner any feedback unless something is painful or uncomfortable. Do not moan or groan or wiggle around because this can be a subtle way of manipulating the active partner into continuing to touch a particular spot. Remaining completely passive will allow your body to experience pleasure more fully. If you become tense, try taking some deep breaths to relax yourself and focus only on the touch.

Feedback

At the end of the exercise, talk openly and honestly with one another about your experience. The exercise will do no good if you lie about your feelings. For instance, please do not tell your partner you enjoyed the experience if you didn't or that you were able to concentrate if you weren't just so that you appear to be doing things correctly.

Most people benefit greatly from giving and receiving feedback after the exercises. This kind of feedback can be the beginning of really honest communication between the couple, establishing trust and openness. Both partners learn to communicate more openly and honestly about what feels good and what doesn't, and they learn what feels good to their partner.

Always do the exercises in a private, quiet environment. Take the phone off the hook, send the children to a baby-sitter or wait until they are in bed at night. Some people prefer to have some easy listening music, but it is really best to do these exercises in silence. It is far too easy to become distracted when there is music, and your intention is to focus on sensations only.

When you give your child (and yourself) the gift of sensuality, you are giving a gift that will last a lifetime. Sensual children are connected to their feelings, their environment, and their bodies and have a far greater chance of connecting with a partner in an authentic, intimate, rewarding way.

In Part I, you learned how to raise a child who is sexually healthy by providing the proper home environment in terms of affection, positive parental messages, proper boundaries, safety, encouragement, and healthy values.

Part II is organized in an entirely different way. It is divided into the normal stages of sexual development that your child will pass through. In this way you can refer for information to the chapter that specifically relates to your child's current age. For example, if your child is already nine years old when you buy the book, you can go right to the chapter addressing issues of that age for help.

While Part I focused on information concerning particular areas of your child's sexuality (body image, values, sensuality), Part II offers specific information on what you can expect in terms of your child's sexual development at each particular age range and offers you help on how to *talk* to your child about his or her age-specific concerns. While Part I focused on *your behavior*, Part II focuses on *your child's behavior*, identifying normal versus abnormal behavior for each age group. And while Part I focused on what you should *do* in order to raise a sexually healthy child, Part II focuses on what you need to *say*—how to talk to your child at each stage of development, how to answer your child's questions, and how to discuss specific issues.

Part II

◆

NORMAL STAGES OF SEXUAL DEVELOPMENT: WHAT TO EXPECT AND WHAT TO TELL YOUR CHILD

INTRODUCTION TO PART II

Children today are changing so rapidly that, frankly, child psychologists and researchers cannot keep up with them. Much of the information gleaned from years of observation and research, information that parents have come to rely on, is now outdated. I will attempt to provide you with information that applies more to kids today, information that is based on the latest research and observation. You may find, therefore, that this information will be different from other books you may have read on childhood development. For example, there have been several books written concerning how and when to talk to your child about sex, depending upon her or his age and stage of development. While these books were written by noted and respected professionals and were accurate based on the information available to them at the time, they may not apply to today's children as much as they once did.

Today's children have grown up in a sex-saturated culture, and it is beginning to take its toll. Because they have been so exposed to sex on television and even in movies that are supposed to be for children, they are far more sexually sophisticated than we were at their age. Today, children as young as four and five years old take an interest in sex, discuss sex, make sexual comments to one another, and even engage in sexual activities that go well beyond normal sex play based on sexual curiosity.

Recent observations at Syracuse University noted that both boys and girls talk about sex between themselves as early as five and six years old, some even younger. Groups of boys age six and seven who were observed while watching television made frequent comments about women's breasts, about wanting to see women naked, and even about intercourse. When given a choice of videos to watch, the most commonly chosen video was a Cindy Crawford workout tape.

Sex is stimulating, even for kids. Those kids who are constantly bombarded with sex on television, in videos, and even in their music are bound to be influenced by it. The atmosphere is so sexually charged that kids can't help but get "hooked" on the excitement even though they are not emotionally or even physically mature enough to handle their sexual feelings.

And children are learning sexual attitudes and values that most parents do not want their children to have. For example, movies like *Roger Rabbit*, *Aladdin*, and *Pocahontas* all portrayed females as voluptuous and sexy. All the young girls ages eight and nine who were observed and interviewed in the Syracuse study stated that the way to get a boy's attention is to be "sexy." Young girls of eight and nine can do a perfect Madonna imitation and are already choosing clothes based on whether they are "sexy" or not.

Television and the movies are clearly influencing children regarding sex. For example, girls are so influenced by movies where women are the aggressors that those girls interviewed said that, in fact, girls are the ones responsible for a couple having sex because they "tempt" boys so much. This is clearly the message that exists in so many teen movies based on the male fantasy of being "overtaken" by a girl.

The incidence of rape and child molestation by other children has increased considerably. While this is most often due to the fact that a child has been sexually abused himself or herself by an adult, it is also suspected that some aggressive sexual behavior on the part of certain children is due to the fact that the child is observing this behavior in adults around him or her. What is referred to as "gangsta" rap portrays women as whores who deserve to be used, abused, and degraded. When a child's role model views sex as a "right" and as a way of dominating others, it is no wonder that so many male children begin to treat female children with such disrespect.

Children are even reaching puberty at a much younger age. It is not uncommon for girls now to begin menstruation as early as nine years old, according to the Syracuse study. Part of the reason for this is undoubtedly better nutrition, but that is only part of the answer. It is strongly suspected that they are beginning menstruation early because they are taking an interest in sex at earlier and earlier ages.

TALKING TO YOUR CHILD ABOUT SEX

It will be helpful to you to become familiar with the stages and behaviors that are considered a part of your child's normal sexual development. My intention here is to focus primarily on psychological development as it relates to sexuality. It is important to remember that each child is unique and will develop at his or her own pace. Some children go through these stages earlier, others later. Never try to force this development; it will occur in its own time.

My desire is to make it possible for you to talk to your child comfortably, rather than assign her or him a book to read (although sometimes this too is recommended). At times I have provided examples of dialogues in order to demonstrate the kinds of questions children ask and the kinds of answers that satisfy them. I have tried to imagine scenarios where both parents are involved in the discussion, where a mother talks to a daughter, a mother talks to a son, or a father talks to a daughter or son. In other words, I have tried to anticipate any configuration—from single parent to coupled parents—in which parents talk to their children.

If your children are to grow up understanding the importance and joys of sexual sharing with a partner of their choice, they need to understand and balance the potential dangers with the probable pleasures of adult sexuality. They need a continuing dialogue with a loving parent regarding all of the sexual issues that they may hear about and misunderstand, as well as the sexual concerns that emerge at each age and developmental stage.

It is up to you to determine what is appropriate and beneficial to pass on to your children and how to share the information. The important factors in this decision are the age of the child and his or her individual characteristics.

A child's age and stage of development are critical factors in providing sexual information because children have age-specific sexual interests and concerns. For example, adolescents from pubescence to sixteen need to be reassured that their sexual development, sexual interest, and desire are natural and normal. They also need detailed information on birth control and sexually transmitted diseases.

The individual characteristics of your child are important too, as you accommodate those differences daily. A curious, confident child can handle more information in a candid, fragmented, or offhand manner than a sensitive, brooding child who personalizes everything he or she learns.

The most important factor in talking to your child about sex is your attitude. If talking about sex causes you to feel extremely embarrassed, you will communicate that embarrassment to your child, and the message the child will receive is that sex is something shameful or dirty. Therefore, it is crucial that you work on your embarrassment regarding sex, look for its roots, and find ways of diminishing it. If you cannot do this no matter how hard you try, you may want your spouse to do most of the sex education of your children (assuming he or she is less embarrassed than you). If you have no spouse, you will need to tell your child that you have a problem being embarrassed about sex, but that you will try to talk to her or him and answer his or her questions. Explain that you do not want her or him to have to suffer from the kind of embarrassment you suffer from. If you cannot talk to your child without conveying the message that sex is dirty and shameful, you may decide simply to provide your child with books or videos.

While sex education is the responsibility of both parents, one parent may be unable or unwilling to take an active role. For example, if your husband refuses to have any part of it, you will need to take it upon yourself to explain sex and love to all the children in your family. Incidentally, it has never been established that girls are better educated by their mothers or boys by their fathers. This is especially good news for single parents who are forced by circumstances to be the one to talk to their opposite-sex child. As mentioned in Chapter Two, sex education is far more than any formal training you may give your child. It is reflected in your behavior with your mate and in your communication with your child on a daily basis.

You will need to communicate to your child that he or she is free to ask you questions about sex *at any time*. This doesn't necessarily mean that you must answer then and there, but you will want to let your child know that he or she asked a very good question and state specifically when you will discuss it. (Children can sometimes ask the most embarrassing questions in front of guests.)

One discussion is not enough, of course. Your first discussion can establish the basics and open the door of trust, permitting the subject to be one of ongoing openness and dialogue.

Probably the most important thing to strive for is a spirit of openness within the family about sexual issues. Children learn more about life—developing attitudes and values—*indirectly* than they do from formal instruction. Therefore, let your children observe you and allow them to overhear and contribute to adult conversations about important topics.

In order to help you with your discussions with your child, I have divided Part II into the four stages of psychosexual development: 1) early childhood sexuality (ages 2–5); 2) the school years (ages 6–9); 3) preadolescence (ages 10–12); and 4) adolescence (ages 13–18). For each stage of development, I describe what your child's developmental tasks will be, and discuss what your child's sexual concerns will be and what type of sexual behavior to expect from your child. Don't be surprised if you find that I list behavior and sexual concerns that you may not think a child that young will be experiencing. For example, other professionals may have suggested you begin talking to your child about sex at around age eight. I suggest you begin at age four or five. Remember, children are constantly being exposed to sex in the media. It is better if they hear the facts from you.

At the end of each chapter, you will find an "Areas for Discussion" section. These sections will require you to go back in time to retrieve childhood memories regarding your own sexual feelings, attitudes, and development. You need to remember what it is like to be a child, a preadolescent, or a teenager in order to appreciate fully what your child is going through at each stage of development.

10

✦

Early Childhood Sexuality (Ages 2–5)

I n Part I we discussed some of the important ingredients in providing your infant and toddler a head start toward healthy sexuality: bonding and nurturing; giving positive messages regarding his or her body, masturbation, and sex; and not overreacting to your child's natural curiosity about his or her body. You will need to continue providing all of these things for your child as he or she gets older. In this chapter I will discuss the preschool years—ages two through five, the years when your child begins to form his or her personality, completes toilet training, continues to learn about sex roles, and begins to ask questions about birth, pregnancy, and genitals.

NORMAL STAGES OF SEXUAL DEVELOPMENT

Children at this age:

- ✦ learn toilet training
- ✦ begin to experience feelings of guilt
- ✦ begin to develop a conscience
- ✦ begin to understand and respect privacy

235

✦ enjoy self-stimulation
✦ discover sex differences
✦ develop sex roles and gender identification
✦ become involved in sex play
✦ may begin to use profanity

TOILET TRAINING

The toilet-training period (usually between two and three years old) is particularly important to your child's sexual development. The reason is simple—the genital areas are in the same area that is used for excretion. If your child develops a positive attitude toward control over excretion, he or she will generalize this positive feeling to the genital area.

Additionally, urinating and excreting are sensual experiences for the child, and this further connects toilet training with sexuality. Toilet training is important to your child's sexual development for still another reason: It is your child's first encounter with self-control, and it is a most difficult task. Toilet training actually involves the mastery of several skills: distinguishing between a full and an empty bladder, recognizing what the sensation is, and, most difficult, acting on the stimulus (that is, going into the bathroom). Mastering this task becomes the child's first triumph over his or her body. Success in this area can develop a young child's self-confidence and self-esteem.

Your emotions around the issue of toilet training will strongly influence your child's attitude and emotions about it. As for developing a toilet-training strategy, remember that the most successful program is also the simplest. Start by praising your child when he or she first begins to discern that he or she has to go to the bathroom. This is true whether the child is able to let you know verbally or whether he or she starts displaying behaviors that indicate he or she has to go to the bathroom. Pour on the praise after each indication that he or she has to make a trip, and lead the child by the hand into the bathroom.

No matter what technique you use to train your child, and there are many to choose from, make sure you only use positive reinforcement. Never punish your child for accidents or for the inability to perform the task. Most professionals recommend a reward system rather than one of punishment or disapproval. Give your child verbal rewards such as: "It's very good to tell me when you need to use the bathroom," or "I'm so proud of you for coming to tell me you needed to go to the bathroom!" Rewards of a small toy or permission to do a favorite activity are also good, but rewards of food are not recommended.

It is important to keep in mind that the ability to control one's bowels is a physical one. The muscles involved in controlling excretion usually develop around the age of two, but for some children this doesn't occur until three. Many parents initiate a toilet-training program long before their child is physically capable of it, and this creates a great deal of frustration for both parent and child. If, despite your efforts, your child is not succeeding, he or she is probably not physically ready. Your child wants to please you and will do so as soon as he or she is able. Be patient.

CHILDREN BEGIN TO EXPERIENCE FEELINGS OF GUILT

Children often begin to develop feelings of guilt around the issue of toilet training. Take special care not to make your child feel he or she is "bad" or that he or she has "failed" when the child does not respond quickly to training. Because your child lacks the ability to understand clearly right from wrong at this age, guilt should be downplayed.

CHILDREN BEGIN TO DEVELOP A CONSCIENCE

During this time, young children begin to develop a conscience. Eager for love and acceptance, the young child looks to his or her parents to approve or disapprove of his or her actions. He or she learns what "no" means and to respect the property of others. This is the time to allow your child to begin making choices. Begin to teach alternatives and set limits and provide information about consequences of behavior.

CHILDREN BEGIN TO UNDERSTAND AND RESPECT PRIVACY

We discussed the issue of privacy extensively in Part I. This is the appropriate age to begin to teach your child that a closed door requires a knock and to respect the property of others. Instruct your child not to go through others' drawers, purses, or wallets. Remember to model these behaviors for your child.

SELF-STIMULATION

Children at this age are interested in their bodies and find pleasure in touching, feeling, and arousing themselves. As we discussed in Part I, too often parents discourage this, and the result is that the child grows up to feel on some level that pleasure through self-stimulation is forbidden, dirty, or even disgusting. These attitudes obviously affect later sexual expression.

If your child engages in masturbatory practices in public or at home in front of other people, simply say, "We don't do that here. People touch themselves and please themselves only when they are alone." Then later, when your child is in his or her bedroom, reinforce the acceptability of self-stimulation with a positive statement such as, "This is the place where it is okay to touch yourself." Children this age are usually satisfied with this explanation. If your child does ask "Why?" you can explain by saying, "Touching yourself is a private activity."

THE DISCOVERY OF SEX DIFFERENCES

It used to be that little girls and little boys began to notice that they were different from one another by the way they dressed, and to some extent this is still true. But today, girls don't always wear dresses, have long hair, or play with dolls, and boys sometimes do wear pink, have long hair, and play with dolls. Whether your child realizes that there are other differences between boys and girls or not, there will come a day when your little girl will suddenly become aware that a boy has a visible appendage to his body that she does not have or your little boy realizes a girl lacks that appendage.

While girls react in different ways, most say something like, "He has more than I have. I want one." A series of doubts may then enter her mind (often unconsciously). She may wonder, "Why didn't Mommy give *me* one of those?" or "Mommy must have punished me by taking it away."

I'm sure you have heard numerous stories about little girls asking Mommy or Daddy to get them a "peenie" or girls trying to urinate while standing up like their dads or big brothers do. But however "cute" such remarks or behavior may seem, to a little girl the worry that there is something wrong with her genitals is serious business and may sometimes color her feelings about being a girl.

It really isn't enough to dismiss a child's concerns with a statement like, "All girls are born like you." Your daughter will need to know through countless ways that being a girl is wonderful, and that all girls and their mommies are built differently from boys and daddies. For example, you might tell your daughter:

✦ Girls are built in a special way that is just right for them. You urinate as your mother does—sitting down—through a small opening for this purpose. A boy urinates from his penis while standing up, just like his daddy.
✦ No girl ever had a penis or lost it in any way.
✦ When a girl gets to be older and becomes a woman, she can grow babies inside of her just as Mommy did.

Far more important is for you to reassure your daughter, now and during her growing years, that she is valued as a girl by both her parents, and that she was very much wanted as a girl by both of you.

This may not convince her for some time because very

young children have a way of clinging to their fantasies, however disturbing they may be. However, with your sensitive understanding of her doubts, and with your help and encouragement, your daughter can gradually come to accept these differences. She will be able to see, particularly through watching and admiring her mother, that each sex has its own special advantages, privileges, and charms.

A little boy has no reason to believe that girls are not constructed in exactly the same way as boys. When your son does find out that a girl has no penis, he may be somewhat stunned and imagine that she was physically hurt in some way. He is likely to wonder, or even come out with a question such as, "What happened to Mary's penis?" It may be quite frightening for him to think, even if unconsciously, "If I'm not careful, something may also happen to *me*."

Some boys react to this fear by reassuring themselves that their penis is still there by handling their penis or even by showing it off. If they're in the throes of toilet training, they may even occasionally fear that their penis could be flushed down the bowl. The sight of handicapped people or damaged toys may intensify these fears.

Sometimes boys are anxious about their genitals because they have been taught to feel guilty about the normal genital play typical of children at this age. Such threats as "If you touch it too much it will fall off" feed right into a small boy's built-in fears.

At this point your son needs reassurance that he cannot lose his penis and that nothing is likely to happen to it or change it. Tell him that girls are built as they are right from the start so that later on they can be mommies, just as someday he will become a daddy. Most of all your son needs to know that both his parents are proud and happy about his being a boy.

Sometimes it is hard to answer your child's first questions about sex differences without feeling some embarrassment. This is especially true if your child asks them in public or if your own questions were cut short with comments like "We don't talk about things like that!" or other admonitions to keep quiet.

Yet, in spite of some initial tension on your part, you can learn to tell your child what she or he is struggling to know.

Not all children ask questions directly during these early years. This is partly due to the fact that some of their worries are only fleeting and barely conscious, or they may feel timid about expressing themselves. And, while some children have the opportunity to observe sex differences directly at this age, not all children have brothers or sisters or playmates of both sexes. They may, however, notice the genitals of a pet or have wondered about the animals at the zoo. Children need to know and understand what these differences mean because they are apt to remain puzzled when no explanation is given. If your child hasn't come out with any questions or statements about sex differences by the time he or she reaches school age, it would be wise to open up the subject yourself.

SEX ROLES AND GENDER IDENTIFICATION

This is the age when your child will learn the most regarding sex roles. By the age of three, your child will more than likely identify with one sex, categorize other people according to their sex, and even come to view certain behaviors as being appropriate to one sex or the other. While you may have gone out of your way to stress the variety of behavior open to each sex, your child will be given the message by other relatives, other children, and even by TV that they should behave in a certain way depending upon what sex they are. (TV teaches children very rigid, inflexible sex roles. Many commercials and programs depict women in a very derogatory manner, making them appear helpless, dependent, and even flaky.) In addition, new research now points to the strong possibility that children may in fact be programmed by genetics to prefer sex-appropriate activities.

The point is that whether you prefer your child to take on traditional sex roles or to learn more flexible ones, you can't change your child's natural awareness of "maleness" and "fe-maleness." Children at this age begin to learn sex-role behaviors, not only from you but from their environment. And to a large extent, healthy sexuality involves developing an awareness of the similarities and differences between the sexes and an appreciation of those differences.

For example, those who are confined to narrow sex roles have difficulties relating to the other sex. They lack understanding of the behavior of members of the other sex and therefore often have little respect for the other's life.

It is important that you understand that each of us has both masculine and feminine characteristics and that a healthy person is one who has integrated the masculine and feminine parts into a whole. Some children go through a phase of having a strong preference for the characteristics and traits of the other sex. For example, girls who prefer masculine activities are often responding to the greater attention paid in the family to "male activities." Often as a result of experiencing a "tomboy" phase, these girls emerge as better integrated and generally more confident.

When a male child prefers feminine activities, it is often because he has no male role models. In this circumstance, just as with the "tomboy" phase in girls, in all likelihood the boy will outgrow these tendencies as he develops friendships at school and in the neighborhood. Parents of males raised in all-female households should try to expose this child to as many masculine activities as possible, but it is no doubt comforting to know that these boys are able to relate well to women and are usually very successful in romantic relationships with the opposite sex.

However, the boy who is extremely feminine and likes only female activities, especially if he prefers female clothes, may be experiencing sexual-identity confusion. This is especially true if this behavior does not stop by the time he enters school. Do not make the mistake of thinking that sexual-identity confusion means homosexuality in a child. In fact, sexual-identity confusion is not a sexual preference, but a serious psychological problem. It means the child is psychologically confused and should be treated by a professional.

If your female child seems to prefer masculine activities and clothes, you probably have less reason to be concerned. Studies have shown that girls often outgrow their "tomboy" phase, and that those girls who do not are more likely to be lesbian (something you have no control over and something that is *not* considered to be a psychological problem) than to have a serious sexual-identity confusion problem. Also, there is far more permission in our society for girls to dress and act masculine, so your daughter isn't as likely to be shunned and teased by her peers as an effeminate male.

Even though your child has learned about his or her *physical* sex differences by age two or three, don't be alarmed if you see your son or daughter mixing up his or her biological sex roles. It is perfectly natural for your son sometimes to want to play Mommy or for your daughter to want to play the role of Daddy. But if at six or seven your child prefers switching roles, it's quite another matter, and you may want either to consult a qualified professional or look for the likely cause of the problem on your own. For example, if you have been longing for a daughter and have been talking about it to friends and family, your little boy may get the idea that girls are preferable to boys, at least in your eyes. Or the natural rejoicing that is going on in the household over your newborn son may give your daughter the idea that because the baby is a different sex the baby is better loved.

Your goal as a parent then should be twofold: 1) to support your child's identification with his or her own sex, and 2) to demonstrate that each sex has many behavior options.

SEX PLAY BETWEEN CHILDREN OF THIS AGE IS PREVALENT

Children who get involved in sex play are just experimenting with what is fun and exciting, and perhaps a bit titillating. They also experiment as a way of trying to make sense out of what they have heard, as a way of creating order for themselves. Although it is disconcerting to find a five-year-old boy examining his five-year-old female friend's "privates," the best thing to do is to keep cool. Instead of becoming upset, remind yourself that it is natural and try to distract the children. (Refer back to Chapter Two, "Laying the Groundwork for Healthy Sexuality.") If you become angry or upset, your child will end up feeling guilty and shameful and will feel you do not understand or approve of his sexual self.

If your child is doing something you don't approve of (it seems too sophisticated for the child's age range or it goes against your values), state your objections and reasons for the objection very gently, while at the same time acknowledging your child's feelings: "I know you are curious, but I'd rather you come to me with your sexual questions," or "I know that what you were doing is exciting, but those things are for when you are older." Remain calm and try to end the conversation on a light note, perhaps with a hug or a pat on the shoulder.

YOUR CHILD MAY BEGIN TO USE PROFANITY

Children of this age often use vulgar language, sometimes to get a rise out of their parents, and other times in order to find out what the words mean. Many children go through a period of "bathroom talk" and utter words that sound amusing to them, with or without knowing their meaning. And by school age, a boy will often make use of slang and "dirty" words to help make himself feel important and popular with his friends.

The trick is not to react too strongly. A strong reaction almost always has the opposite effect of what you hope for. Because of the charm of the forbidden, the unmentionable words may become exciting; or they may go underground and be used in secret. It is best simply to correct your child just as you'd correct his or her bad manners. Calmly let the child know that you know the meaning of the words he or she used, but that maybe *he* or *she* doesn't; then explain matter-of-factly. Your child should know that there are words he or she shouldn't use around you because you don't like them and your friends don't like them. Your child will more than likely soon become bored with this phase.

AREAS FOR DISCUSSION: WHAT YOUR PRESCHOOLER NEEDS TO KNOW ABOUT SEX

CHILDREN AT THIS AGE ARE FILLED WITH CURIOSITY

This is the age when your child will be full of questions. His or her "sexual" concerns will be mostly focused on where babies come from and the differences between boys and girls. Give your child enough information to satisfy his or her healthy curiosity, but not more than he or she can understand. This is the time to answer questions about pregnancy, birth, and breast-feeding with brief but honest answers that you can elaborate on as time goes by.

In addition, five-year-olds will hear words on TV such as *rape, molestation,* and *AIDS.* It is important to explain in a basic way what these words mean. Now is the time to explain sexual abuse, avoiding strangers, inappropriate touching, and yes, even sexually transmitted disease. By allowing your child to ask these questions, you lay the foundation for future discussions about sexuality. Your child should know he or she can always come to you with questions. Refer back to Part I for tips on how to conduct these discussions.

NAMING BODY PARTS

One of the first and most important kinds of sexual information you can provide for your child is teaching your toddler the names of his or her body parts. At the same age that you begin identifying and teaching the names of legs and arms, eyes and ears, you can include nipples, vagina, penis, testicles, and anus. Just as you don't find a substitute name for shoulder or neck, there is no reason to use a substitute word for penis or vagina. A sexually healthy child takes pride in all parts of his or her body and learns that all parts of the body are miraculous and should be used wisely and well.

Children who are two and under are satisfied with names,

but as children become more verbal they like to know what these organs do. Just as you tell them that eyes are for seeing and ears are for hearing, you will need to say that penises are for urinating and making babies, vaginas are for urinating and having babies, nipples (in girls) are for milk, and anuses are for bowel movements. By the time your child is approximately four years old, he or she should know these organs and their function.

WHERE BABIES COME FROM

Children at this age need simple answers to their questions. They don't need you to elaborate or to give them more information than they can absorb. For example, when your child asks you, "Mommy, where do babies come from?" or "Where did I come from?" you can give an uncomplicated but *correct* answer such as:

"A tiny seed called a sperm from Daddy met a tiny egg called an ovum inside me. That's how you got started. Then you grew and grew inside my uterus for nine months. Then you were born."

If your child asks, "How was I born?" simply state, "You came out through Mommy's vagina."

Since you are going to be helping your child to name all his or her body parts, including genitals, use the proper names for the reproductive system as well. The child doesn't have to remember these names, of course, but you want to give him or her accurate information instead of fantasies like "the stork" or the "cabbage patch."

By now your child's basic sexual orientation is set in place, his or her sense of maleness or femaleness is clear, he or she has accomplished the major task of toilet training, and he or she is beginning to understand the concept of privacy. A lot has happened in very little time!

Remember that at every stage of development your child needs constant reassurance from you that he or she is loved, accepted, and safe. Couples need to model affection and acceptance by openly expressing your love and caring for one another. And positive interactions between all members of the family (parents, siblings, grandparents) will contribute to your child's sense of comfort and safety.

PARENTAL ISSUE: SEXUAL HISTORY

Your sexual history affects what you teach and model for your children as much as your sexual beliefs and values. Reach back into your memory to try to recapture those events in your life that shaped your sexuality. This process may be difficult at times and may bring up strong emotions that you may have buried.

Start with the earliest memories you have of being a child. Go back to infancy if you can. Try to remember who held you and did not hold you. Did your mother and father take you into their bed for cuddling? Try to remember who dressed you as a child and whether your clothes reflected whether you were a boy or girl. Were your toilet-training experiences mostly positive or mostly negative? Was there a respect for personal privacy in your household? Were you often praised for how pretty or how cute you looked? Who bathed you? Was it the parent of the same sex?

After you have spent some time remembering, you may find it rewarding to share some or all of your memories with your partner (if you have one). Talking with your partner about your own childhood sexual experiences should make it easier to find an opportunity to initiate a similar discussion with your child.

11

◆

The School Years (Ages 6–9)

Although this period is often referred to as the "latency" period, your child will nevertheless continue progressing toward sexual development. He or she will continue to gather information, experiment with his or her own sexuality, observe with great interest the sexuality of others, and from these observations form impressions about sexuality. This is the time when children can learn that their parents are the ones to turn to for sexual information, guidelines, and values. This is also the time when your child will begin to connect with other people outside of the home in important ways, bringing up the issues of parental jealousy, peer pressure, normal sexual play among children, and children being introduced to sex by older, more experienced children.

NORMAL STAGES OF SEXUAL DEVELOPMENT

Children at this age will:

✦ experience relationships outside the family

✦ experiment with homosexual sexuality
✦ sometimes develop romantic feelings for parents

YOUR CHILD WILL EXPERIENCE RELATIONSHIPS OUTSIDE THE FAMILY

As your child starts school, he or she will meet many new people and make new friends. Suddenly teachers seem to know as much as Mommy and Daddy. Friends become increasingly important, as do older siblings. You will begin to hear more statements like "Tiffany's mother lets her wear lipstick, why can't I?" Parental authority begins to crumble, and it will be common to hear "Yeah, well, Miss Flanders says . . ." Be careful not to be jealous of your child's new attachment to a favorite teacher, a coach, or other authority figures. This is a necessary and important attachment, one on which future attachments will depend. If you understand and encourage your child's praise and idolizing of the newest "role model," then he or she will feel it is okay to care about other people in addition to you. When parents become insecure ("Don't you love me anymore?") or react with jealousy ("All you ever talk about is Miss Flanders"), their child quickly receives the message that it is not okay to form attachments and friendships with others—that it is somehow disloyal to do so.

Encourage your child to become more independent. Whether you want it to happen or not, your child will be expanding his or her sources of information. This is also the time when your child will be exposed to things that you probably wouldn't allow, such as more explicit TV shows and movies at his or her friends' houses.

Children at this age will also be exposed to information from their peers and siblings. There is little you can do to prevent "premature" learning, so you will need to establish sound values and provide your child with accurate information and let him or her know that you are there if he or she ever needs clarification.

CHILDREN WILL EXPERIMENT WITH HOMOSEXUAL SEXUALITY

Homosexual experiences among children are extremely common and completely normal and natural. If you find your child involved in a homosexual activity such as mutual touching, remember this and don't overreact. The chances are that the incident means absolutely nothing. (Caution: anal or oral sex at this age is *not* normal and is likely to be a symptom of previous sexual abuse.) Calmly tell the children to put on their clothes and come out for a talk. Tell them that although they were enjoying themselves, these kinds of activities are not allowed for children. Forty-six percent of the male population in our nation (and other Western nations) report at least one homosexual experience in their lifetime. Many men and women will have several homosexual experiences and still have a heterosexual preference.

CHILDREN WILL SOMETIMES DEVELOP ROMANTIC FEELINGS FOR PARENTS

It is common for your child to develop "romantic" feelings toward the opposite-sex parent. These feelings are often triggered by watching his or her parents be affectionate with one another. The reason for this reaction is that children at this age have already identified with the same-sex parent, and thus they want to love the other-sex parent in the same way as the same-sex parent does.

These romantic attachments are normal and usually occur after the age of four. But unless you make it clear to your child that he or she is not ever going to be the object of your romantic affection, the attachment can last well into your child's teens. Therefore, you will need to firmly discourage your child's romantic ideas.

For example, if your son tells you he is going to marry you when he grows up, don't just go along with it. Explain that parents don't marry their children and that you already have a spouse (if you do). Tell him that you love him in a different way than you love your spouse and that one day he will grow up and fall in love with someone just like you did with his father.

Many single parents encounter another problem. Often, when they begin to date once again, they discover that their child feels threatened, jealous, and angry that she or he now has to share her or his parent with someone else.

These parents often feel terribly conflicted. On the one hand, they want to begin dating once again, but on the other, they don't want to cause their child pain. Many single parents already feel guilty over putting their child through a divorce, and so they desperately try to make their child's life as easy as possible.

While it is understandable that you will want to be sensitive to your child's feelings, it is vitally important that you do not allow your child to dictate whom you will date or to control your romantic relationships in any way.

Instead, talk to your child about the situation, making certain that you acknowledge your child's feelings of jealousy, threat, or anger. An appropriate statement might be: "I understand that you feel Thomas is going to take me away from you, but no one can do that." Then explain that you will always love your child and that the love a parent has for a child is very different from the kind of love a woman has for a man. This kind of conversation will help your child understand and eventually accept your need for a romantic relationship with another grown-up.

AREAS FOR DISCUSSION

CONTINUE TEACHING THE BASIC FACTS OF LIFE

Just because your child is more preoccupied with friendships and activities, doesn't mean he or she has lost interest in his or her body and bodily functions. TV, videos, and friends' conversations will constantly expose your child to sexual material, so you must continue to provide him or her with information, whether he or she asks or not.

Although you have been talking to your child about sex all during his or her childhood, the very best time to discuss sex is the ages from seven to nine. At these ages, children are the most open to what you have to say. This is also before the age when they are primarily influenced by their peers.

Seven or eight may seem like a young age for some of the discussions listed below, but it is the right age for two very important reasons: 1) To wait longer runs the risk (if not the strong possibility) that your child will learn of reproduction and sex from other children; 2) eight years old is a natural and curious age when children can understand in a sweet, uncynical way.

The questions that will continue to perplex your child center around the following subjects:

+ Why do I have a penis?
+ Why do I have a vagina?
+ How are babies made?
+ Do you make a baby every time?
+ Do you have to be married to have a baby?

These questions are not all that different from the ones asked when he or she was younger. What is different is that now the answers need to be fuller and more detailed because your child can now understand more and even compare information with friends. It doesn't matter who does the explaining, Mom or Dad. Ideally, you can answer your child's questions together, but because both parents are seldom at home when the questions are asked, and because you want to answer your child's questions promptly, it will more than likely be only one of you who will answer the questions. Postponing the discussion until you are both at home tends to make a big deal out of something that should be seen as natural.

Offer more than just reproductive information when answering questions. Don't ignore the most important aspects of sexuality—feelings associated with sex (love, intimacy), male and female roles, differences and similarities between men and women, values, guidelines, and your own personal experiences. Children need to know this kind of information as much as reproductive information.

It is also important to realize that children of this age understand best what is *concrete*, meaning what they can see, feel, touch, and taste. Therefore, when you answer a child's question or have a discussion with your child, try to be as explicit as possible. The following discussion about how a woman becomes pregnant is a good example:

CHILD: How does a woman become pregnant?
PARENT: The male inserts his penis into the female's vagina. Sperm are ejaculated from the male into the vagina during sexual intercourse, and they swim up the vagina and into the fallopian tubes. If an egg has been released and swept into one of the fallopian tubes, a sperm can unite with it and fertilize it—and the female can become pregnant. A fertilized egg plants itself inside the lining of the uterus, grows inside the uterus, and eventually develops into a baby.
CHILD: Does a woman have to be married to get pregnant?
PARENT: No, she can get pregnant any time she has intercourse. Many women have sex without being married.

It is entirely appropriate for you to begin talking about love and intimacy to children this age without overwhelming them or talking over their heads. You can talk about how some people "fall in love" with one another and how others "grow" into love, perhaps by being close friends first. Talk about how over time two people may choose to express their love through sexuality. You can share your views concerning the appropriateness of premarital sex, birth control, and so on, but remember to bring in the human factor. For example: "I believe that sex is better when two people are committed to one another because then there is trust and security within the relationship.

Both partners can relax more, and then sex can enhance the love that is already there."

COUNTERACTING PEER PRESSURE AND MISINFORMATION

Children who receive accurate information from their parents will not be as influenced by the many myths and misconceptions that their peer groups pass along. The time to initiate an open communication is during the child's early school years. This means that parents need to answer each and every question their child poses honestly and openly and to realize that if a child is curious enough to pose a question, then he or she is old enough to know the answer.

The more you are able to communicate freely with your child about sexuality, the more you will be able to influence his or her development. Since your child knows how you feel about important issues, he or she will be more likely to adopt your values or at least to see your point of view. And he or she will also be more likely to turn to you for guidance and support. In addition, you will be more likely to know what is going on in your child's life and how he or she is feeling. This in turn will allow you to offer the kind of support and guidance he or she needs at the time.

WHAT IS NORMAL SEX PLAY?

It used to be that the only thing parents needed to worry about with children during the so-called latency period was masturbation and sex play. But today, many children are becoming sexually active before they even reach sexual maturity. Others are constantly having to withstand pressure from older or more experienced children. And some are even being coerced into sexual activity by children who have been introduced to sex too early or have been sexually molested.

As I've stated earlier, sexual curiosity is normal in children. All children explore their own bodies, and to some extent, they may engage in visual or even manual exploration of another child's body. This is one way that children discover sexual differences or verify what they have been told by their parents or others about the differences between boys and girls. But often children may appear to consent even though they actually do not. In many instances, what appears to be consent may actually be only passive consent or the inability to make a rational decision because of limited cognitive skills and life experiences.

Sexual contact between children is often misunderstood as being just normal sex play. But normal sex play and exploration occurs *only* between those of a similar age, sexual experience, and power. For example, "playing doctor" between consenting age-peers is likely to represent normal sexual experimentation, while sexual activity between a young child and an adolescent represents sexual abuse.

Determining the level of experience of your child's friends will be difficult but not impossible. Pay attention to the dress, behavior, and language of your child's friends. If one of your child's friends dresses in a way that you consider too old, too sexy, or inappropriate for his or her age; if he or she frequently grabs his or her crotch, talks incessantly about penises or breasts, or uses sexually derogatory or vulgar language, this may indicate that he or she has more sexual experience than your child, or at the very least that the child is too mature for your child. If you know for a fact that one of your child's friends has been sexually abused, you need to be aware of the strong possibility that this child may pass on sexual behaviors to your child. While you may decide to allow your child to continue to play with a precocious, more experienced, or abused child, you will need to monitor their activities closely. This means not allowing them to play alone and unsupervised for long periods of time and not allowing them to play alone in your child's room with the door closed.

Only under certain special circumstances is sexual activity between children *not* sexual abuse:

1. The children are approximately the same age.
2. They each have equal power, both with each other and

in the family if they are related. This rules out any situation where one child is in charge of another or has any authority over the other. It also rules out any sexuality between an older male child and a female child even one year younger, since males generally have more power in our society than females.

3. There is no betrayal of trust between them. This would be possible only if they were of the same age and each had equal power. For example, a younger child has a certain amount of trust in an older child, especially if it is an older sibling, a baby-sitter, or a group leader. If the person in authority misuses this trust, the child feels betrayed in an extremely profound way—sometimes causing her or him to mistrust all authority figures in the future.

4. There is no coercion or physical force.

5. The sexual play is the result of natural curiosity, exploration, and mutual sexual naiveté. This is not the case when an older or more experienced child "teaches" the younger one what he or she has learned. In fact, what is generally going on here is that the more experienced child may have been sexually abused and is reenacting the sexual abuse he or she suffered by repeating the cycle of abuse and violence.

6. The children are not traumatized by disapproving parents who may "catch them in the act."

TALKING TO YOUR CHILD ABOUT AIDS

Your child may ask you about AIDS if he or she sees a TV program about it or hears people discussing it. Prepubescent children are not in danger of contracting AIDS. Children from seven to approximately ten or twelve need to be reassured that they are not at risk. Tell your child that the children who have AIDS were infected before they were born because their mother or father had AIDS (here's your chance to reinforce your child's knowledge about conception and gestation) or because they received a blood transfusion before donated blood was tested for AIDS. Explain that the AIDS virus is carried in the blood and that some people, who didn't even know they had AIDS, donated blood to help others. Blood transfusions are now tested and safe.

Children need to know that having AIDS does not mean you are a bad person. Reassure them that children who have AIDS are not contagious like boys and girls who have a cold, chicken pox, or measles, because you can only get AIDS if the virus gets into your blood. They can be a friend to a child with AIDS because you don't get AIDS from casual contact, touching toys or pencils or crayons, or from coughing or sneezing.

If they ask, you can also explain that doctors and nurses use sterile disposable needles when they give shots. This is also your chance to talk about the dangers of recreational intravenous drug use. Remember, though, that children at this age understand things they can see, hear, touch, taste, and smell. Germs and viruses are hard concepts to grasp.

We would hope that children will be influenced more by their parents than by the messages they receive in movies, on television, and in music. But in order for this to be true, parents need to begin talking to their children about sex at earlier and earlier ages.

Just because your child has been exposed to sex, or rather *overexposed*, it does not mean that he or she knows all there is to know. There is still a great deal of misinformation being passed on to children, and as I mentioned earlier, there are certainly a lot of inappropriate attitudes about sex being introduced to your child. Therefore, your child needs you to be the one to provide him or her with *accurate* information about sex, to provide him or her with the appropriate values regarding sex, and to teach him or her appropriate sexual behavior.

PARENTAL ISSUES: CHILDHOOD MEMORIES

YOUR FIRST SEXUAL CONTACT WITH ANOTHER PERSON

Aside from the messages you received from your family, your peers, and society in general about sex, there were other experiences that you had as a child that strongly affected your sexuality. Most notably, your first sexual contact with another person is one of the most significant events influencing your sexuality. Hopefully, your first sexual experience was either a positive or neutral one, not one that would elicit tremendous shame or fear. If the person who introduced you to sex was another child, the chances are that the experience may have been one of innocent exploration and curiosity and one that left you with positive feelings.

How do you feel when you think of your first sexual experience with someone else? No matter how innocent, no matter how young you were, you probably remember the moment quite vividly and probably have strong feelings about it.

Childhood is full of embarrassing experiences, but the ones involving our genitals and our sexuality can be especially humiliating. Children are extremely preoccupied with "fitting in," so they will often go along with other children, even when they don't really want to. Sex is a very private matter, for children as well as adults, and being introduced to it, even by another child, is fraught with potential embarrassment. If the feeling of shame or humiliation was significant enough, it may follow the child into adulthood, coloring her or his adult sexual relationships.

WHEN YOUR FIRST SEXUAL EXPERIENCE WAS SEXUAL ABUSE

While many do not recognize it as such, often our first sexual experience was sexual abuse. Thousands upon thousands of children are sexually abused every year by relatives, caretakers, and other children. One of the reasons why so many victims of child sexual abuse do not recognize they were indeed abused is that many people believe they were willing participants when, in fact, they were being coerced or manipulated by an older, more experienced person, whether it be a child or an adult.

♦

EXERCISE

Your First Sexual Experiences

Spend some time remembering your first experiences with masturbation:

✦ Do you remember exploring your own body?

✦ How old were you when you first began to masturbate?

✦ Were you ever caught or found out?

✦ How were you made to feel?

✦ Were you punished or scolded? Would you have felt differently if you hadn't been made to feel that what you were doing was wicked, bad, or dirty?

Now spend some time remembering your first experiences with sexual exploration and sexual play. Were they positive or shame-filled?

✦ Who first introduced you to sex?

✦ Did you play "doctor" or look at the genital areas of someone of the opposite sex?

✦ How old were you and how old was this person? Do you now believe you were coerced? Was the experience positive or negative?

✦ Were you ever caught? If so, what happened?

✦ How do you think these early experiences with sex affected your later sexual development?

♦

Even though the changes your child experiences from ages six to eight are more internal than external, these are very important years. Although sexual interest and sexual development are not as *observable* during this so-called latency period, they are nevertheless present. While it is during this phase that their interest in sexuality can sometimes take a backseat for a while, children of this age are still very inquisitive about sex and continue developing their understanding of sexuality—they just do it rather quietly.

Because there is no interference from great emotional fluctuation due to hormonal imbalance, such as teens will experience in puberty, this is a great time for sex education and a time when the foundations for more complex issues of sexuality can be laid.

12

◆

Reaching Sexual Maturity—The Preadolescent Stage (Ages 10–12)

This is a time of transition for your child. She or he is not quite a teen and no longer a little child. Changes have been gradual over the past few years, but now your child will go through another important growth spurt. During these developing years, parents and preteens alike need to be preparing for the all-important adolescent years, easily the most significant ones of a child's sexual development and usually the most difficult for both parents and teens. Preteens need to be prepared for what to expect in regard to their own sexual development, particularly as they will inevitably begin to experiment to varying degrees with their sexuality. Those children who have been prepared for puberty tend to adjust to the changes far more easily than those who have not been prepared, both in terms of being more accepting of the changes and being more confident that the changes will be positive.

As soon as their bodies begin to develop, preteens know that they will never be the same. Some look forward to these changes, while others don't. Because of a lack of adequate information about sex and the way the body reacts to sexual stimulation, many preteens become upset and fearful about their body's reactions.

Children must be prepared for puberty well in advance—girls for the onset of menstruation, boys for nocturnal emissions—so that these events do not come as traumatic surprises. In addition, girls and boys should be informed fully of the developments affecting the opposite sex.

NORMAL STAGES OF SEXUAL DEVELOPMENT

Preadolescents:

+ increase masturbation
+ need help coping with different rates of maturation
+ need opportunities to relate to the opposite sex

PREADOLESCENTS INCREASE MASTURBATION

In Chapter Two we discussed making sure that you don't give your child negative messages about masturbation by scolding or making the child feel she or he is doing something wrong. Most parents feel that the best thing to do is just to ignore the issue completely, thinking this is appropriate given the fact that masturbation is a private and personal matter. But children know that it is only the taboo subjects that are not discussed. Therefore, when parents ignore the subject, they are in fact communicating a negative attitude.

Healthy masturbation practices are the foundation on which a satisfying sexual life is built, and because of this it is vitally important that children develop a healthy attitude concerning it. Self-stimulation familiarizes children with their own body and its sexual response. Only by knowing their body can they pass on the information of what pleases them to their partners.

And so you will need to talk with your child openly about masturbation, and the best time for such a discussion is when he or she is between the ages of nine and twelve, the ages when she or he will be most likely to begin to masturbate on a regular basis. Begin the conversation by asking if he or she knows what masturbation is. If your child says he or she doesn't (and he or she may say this even if he or she does), explain to the child that masturbation is touching yourself, especially the genital area, in a way that is both pleasurable and exciting. Tell your child that if he or she already does this it is good because masturbation is the first way you learn about your body and what feels good. Also tell your child that if he or she doesn't already masturbate, he or she may soon begin to feel like it and that this is natural and healthy.

On the other hand, some parents may be concerned that their child is masturbating excessively. Excessive masturbation (more than two to three times a day) is nearly always a sign that a child is troubled emotionally and needs some help. Teach your child that self-stimulation is a positive avenue of sexual pleasure and that those who know how to please themselves sexually have more fulfilling sexual relations with others. Once it is clear to your child that masturbation is normal and healthy, he or she will not feel guilty and thus will be much less likely to become a compulsive masturbator. It is often guilt that creates the energy for compulsive masturbation.

If your child understands that masturbation is normal and healthy, but still continues to masturbate compulsively, it may be that he or she is using masturbation as a pressure release, a way of trying to find some relief from some of his or her anxieties and tensions. The child may not have found a better way of solving his or her problems and seeks escape from them in this way. If this seems to be the case, try to find out the following:

✦ Does he or she feel that more attention and affection are going to a younger or older brother or sister?
✦ Are there plenty of opportunities for her or him to find adventure, interest, excitement, and healthy release for her or his energies?
✦ Is he or she lonely? Is he or she having trouble making friends?
✦ Is she or he getting a sense of satisfaction and achievement from studies, from the mastery of skills?

✦ Is too much being expected of him or her, or is the child constantly being criticized instead of praised?

Let your child know that self-gratification should not be his or her only satisfaction or release. Try to interest her or him more in the outside world. Let your child know that her or his main satisfactions should come from personal relationships and achievements.

If your child still remains troubled and preoccupied with masturbation after you have tried all these measures—and have let ample time go by to see what happens—then it may be time to seek professional help. It is possible, for example, that your child may have been sexually abused. And remember, whatever you do to help your child's total emotional adjustment helps his or her sexual adjustment as well.

PREADOLESCENTS NEED HELP COPING WITH DIFFERENT RATES OF MATURATION

The changes of puberty occur gradually, not at a single point in time. Pubescence begins for females between the ages of nine and twelve, and menarche usually occurs between eleven and fourteen. Puberty begins later for boys, and there is a great variance as to age. It usually begins at ten or eleven and lasts much longer, usually until the age of fifteen or sixteen.

Because the rate of maturation is an individual one, preadolescents need to be continually reassured that they are normal. Preteens often worry that they are not growing or developing as fast as their friends. "Late bloomers" need reassurance that they will eventually develop even though they are not following the growth patterns of their peers. And "early bloomers" need to be prepared to deal with all the extra attention their early development is bound to attract. Both late bloomers and early bloomers need to be taught how to deal with teasing from their peers.

Girls will generally develop about two years ahead of boys. This should be explained to both boys and girls.

PREADOLESCENTS NEED OPPORTUNITIES TO RELATE TO THE OPPOSITE SEX

At this age, social interaction becomes all-consuming. It is common for a preteen to have frequent romantic crushes and to experiment with boy-girl relationships. The stress of these early experiments often brings about tension, embarrassment, and confusion.

Encourage your child to invite others to your home when you are there. This will give you the chance to see the kinds of friends your child is making, and it will give your child the opportunity to meet other children in a safe place.

This is also the time to reteach the equality of the sexes and the appreciation of differences in male and female attitudes.

AREAS FOR DISCUSSION

The junior high school period is probably the clearest demarcation between childhood and adolescence, even though a group of chronological peers at this age is a study in disparity. The new school/social setting prompts even the youngest to strive for the pseudo-adult facade that is to be the hallmark of the next few years. It is at this age when they are feeling their most mature and intellectual selves that preadolescents will agree to discuss sexual topics with adults.

During this time your child may become more modest, and the need for privacy may take on a new importance. Sexual curiosity at this age will probably stem from what the child sees going on around her or him, what she or he hears others say, or what she or her views on TV. Preadolescents are curious about sex, but remain somewhat detached in their interest. Most of their interest involves what is going on with others, what others are doing sexually—not so much themselves— although they are capable of masturbating to orgasm.

Preadolescents should be provided with detailed information

regarding puberty, masturbation, pregnancy, childbirth, sexual intercourse, and male and female anatomy. They need clear, positive, and in-depth explanations using the correct terminology about all of the following:

✦ Male and female sexual responses
✦ The purposes and causes of vaginal lubrication, erection, and wet dreams
✦ How a child is conceived
✦ What circumcision is and why it is performed
✦ Proper menstrual hygiene and various types of feminine products

As a parent, your most important task with the early teen is to prepare your son or daughter to look forward to the rewards of sexual sharing despite our increasingly negative sociosexual climate. Instead of undermining the joys of sexual intimacy by instilling doubt, fear, and guilt, help your early teen by acknowledging that sexual sharing is a healthy, pleasurable human experience, and by emphasizing that his or her sexual choices will have a significant impact (good or bad) on his or her own life, the lives of others, and society at large.

Provide age-appropriate books on human sexuality including materials on the history of sex, the politics of sex, sex and religion, sexual art, and sexual health. Junior high school students like to contemplate and discuss similarities and differences of topics that interest them.

TEACHING ABOUT BODILY CHANGES

All of the physical changes as well as the emotional mood swings of puberty should be carefully discussed with your preteen. The lists below summarize the information you should know about the development of your preteen. They also can be used in discussing and preparing your preteen for the changes that will soon occur in her or him and with her or his peers. Boys and girls not only have different sexual development, but they develop at different ages. Boys need to know what is happening to girls, and girls who know about boys' development do much better understanding and managing male sexuality.

Preteens' development generally falls into four categories:

✦ General physical development, including all body development except for the sexual organs
✦ Sexual physical development, including sexual organs and secondary sexual development (like pubic hair)
✦ Emotional development, including emotional changes
✦ Social development, including all social interactions, mostly with peers but also with adults

What to Expect: Boys Ages Nine to Twelve

General physical development

✦ Taller, broader growth and development of more muscles and greater strength
✦ Breast swelling and tenderness
✦ More perspiration, body odor
✦ Oilier hair and skin
✦ Hair growth on arms and legs, underarms, and development of a beard
✦ Pimples and possible acne
✦ Voice changes

Sexual physical development

✦ More erections
✦ Pubic hair develops (starts out straight, becomes kinkier)
✦ Penis grows
✦ Scrotum enlarges, becomes more wrinkled, looser, and baggier
✦ Ejaculation begins
✦ Nocturnal emissions begin
✦ Masturbation increases (and sexual fantasies develop)

Emotional development

- ✦ Stronger sexual feelings
- ✦ Anxiety about sexual fantasies and masturbation
- ✦ Stronger interest in girls (yet may attempt to hide it)
- ✦ Sexual interest in girls
- ✦ Self-image becomes shaky (sensitivity to mistakes, fears, and perceived "failures")
- ✦ Struggle to gain control of self, be manly
- ✦ Defensiveness

Social development

- ✦ Interest in opposite sex
- ✦ Struggle to learn social skills (conversation, dancing, dating, and "party" behavior)
- ✦ Focus on appearing "manly" socially, identification with social male stereotypes (macho, strong-silent type, protective)
- ✦ Overreaction to mistakes and perceived "failures" in peer relations
- ✦ Internal pressure felt to achieve in some special field that he can identify as "his" (a sport, fixing cars, a hobby)
- ✦ Growing interest in TV, videos (especially adventure, action, drama, sports, and sexy commercials)
- ✦ Pressure felt to achieve scholastically, especially in competition with girls
- ✦ Avoidance of closeness, touching, and nudity, greater modesty
- ✦ Membership in secret clubs or gangs

What to Expect: Girls Ages Nine to Twelve

General physical development

- ✦ Growth spurts (earlier than for boys, taller than boys for about two years)
- ✦ Temporary weight gain (three to five pounds)
- ✦ Rounding and filling out of hips, buttocks, thighs, and shoulders

- Breast development, swelling and tenderness of breasts and extremities
- Tenderness and bloating of abdomen, backaches
- More perspiration, body odor
- Increasing body hair, including growth of underarm hair, possible fuzzy hair on lips
- Pimples, possible acne
- Change in vaginal discharge
- Increased appetite and thirst
- Alternation of extra energy and lack of energy
- Onset of menstruation

Sexual physical development

- Growing vulva
- Fluids begin to appear in vulva area and vagina
- Masturbation increases
- Onset of sexual fantasies
- Pubic hair (starts straight, becomes more kinky)
- Clitoral stimulation more sexually arousing

Emotional development

- Stronger sexual feelings
- Increased sensitivity to mistakes, fears, perceived "failures"
- Mood shifts
- Tension and anxiety
- Interest in boys
- Concentration varies (may increase and/or decrease)
- Irritability
- Self-image shaky
- Defensiveness

Social development

- Avoidance of closeness, nudity, and touch
- Bursts of social activity (dancing, parties, increased interest in group activities)
- More "womanly" social appearance and identification with social sex stereotypes (caretaker, seductress)

- ✦ Intense reaction to failures, mistakes, and rejection in social peer relations
- ✦ Higher scholastic achievement than boys
- ✦ More interest in and awareness of love stories and events like marriage and birth
- ✦ Exposure to public sex (TV, videos, movies, advertisements, etc.)
- ✦ Interest in opposite sex

PREPARING FOR BODILY CHANGES

This stage of development gives you the opportunity to anticipate your child's need for information and guidance. You have a head start if you can get in there ahead of the crisis. Both fathers and mothers should talk openly to their sons and daughters about the sexual maturation process for both males and females. It is even possible to teach your female and male children about sex at the same time. What is important is that you take the shame and secrecy out of sex and that you teach sexuality in a lighthearted, open manner.

Again, you cannot control what your child will hear, when she or he will hear it, or how she or he will construe the meaning of what is heard. By bringing up the subject of sex, however, you get a chance to learn what your child has heard and how he or she interprets it. And he or she gets the message that you are an accepting resource for sexual information. In this way you may be able to reduce some of his or her experimentation outside the house, or at least encourage him or her to conduct those experiments with more information and understanding.

Purchasing some books on teaching children about sex and deliberately leaving them around the house where your preteen can find them is a good way of educating your child. In this way he or she can read the book in privacy without risking embarrassment. Later on, you can casually ask your child if he or she found the book, ask how he or she liked it, and if he or she has any questions.

One of the best ways to build trust is with self-revelation. If you volunteer your secrets to your child, you are showing that you trust her or him, and this in turn will help your child return that trust. Make sure you do not push your child for revelation and that your own is in good taste.

TALKING ABOUT MENSTRUATION

It is important to remember that each female has her own timetable concerning menstruation. Some begin as young as nine years old, some don't begin until sixteen. Since more and more girls are starting menstruation at nine, it seems like a good time to prepare them. How much does your daughter need to know at nine? Basically, a detailed description of why menstruation occurs, when it is likely to occur, and how it will affect her. The following is a good example of such a conversation between mother and daughter:

MOTHER: Remember when you asked me how babies were born? I told you that a man inserts his penis into the woman's vagina and then the man ejaculates sperm into the vagina that then travel up to the uterus. If the woman has an egg in her uterus that meets with the sperm, then a baby can get started. Do you remember that?

DAUGHTER: Yes.

MOTHER: Now I think you are old enough to hear the rest of the story. If the egg and the sperm meet and the egg is fertilized, then your body prepares to take care of this fertilized egg and builds a kind of nest for it in the uterus so that the baby will grow. But if the egg is not fertilized, then the thick lining of the uterus, which grew in order to protect the egg, flows out of the woman's body, sort of like urine, only it comes in the form of blood. It takes anywhere from five to seven days to stop, and it happens once a month. This is called menstruation or starting your period. You've probably heard of that phrase. I'm telling you all this because your body is beginning to mature, and you might begin to menstruate soon. It might happen when you are nine or it might not happen until much later. I want you to know about it so that if you find your panties bloody one day, you won't be frightened. You will know that it is normal—that it is part of growing up.

DAUGHTER: Is that when I will start to wear a tampon?

MOTHER: Yes, or you may prefer to wear a pad. I'll show you where I keep both of them later on, and you can choose.

DAUGHTER: Can people tell if you are having your period?

MOTHER: No, no one can tell. There is nothing dirty or secret about having a period. Every woman does it. I just got over my period.

DAUGHTER: I didn't know that you had one.

MOTHER: Yes, I am only in my forties. Some women continue having their period until they are in their late fifties.

This is a lot of information to try to relay in one sitting. Another good time to repeat the information is when one of your daughter's friends starts her period or when the subject comes up some other way. This is a natural way to reintroduce the information so that your daughter is fully prepared and not embarrassed when her time comes.

If you attempt to talk to your daughter about menstruation and she doesn't seem receptive, don't get discouraged. Just wait for another time and try again. You may want to show her a pad and tampon and ask her if she knows what they are and what they are for.

EXPLAINING NOCTURNAL EMISSIONS

In much the same way that you will need to explain menstruation to your daughter, around the age of ten you will need to explain nocturnal emissions to your son. Mothers can explain this to their son if there is no father or father figure around to do it. Again, I offer a sample conversation, this time between a father and son:

FATHER: Soon you will begin to have what is called nocturnal emissions or "wet dreams." When you have a dream that is very sexually exciting, you will get an erection, and you may ejaculate even though you are still asleep. This is perfectly natural and normal, and it happens to every growing boy. I expect it will happen to you somewhere between eleven and fifteen. I want you to know about it ahead of time so that you won't be frightened, worried, or embarrassed.

SON: Yeah, I heard about that. Does it get all over the sheets?

FATHER: It can. When it happens, you can put them into the hamper and change your sheets.

SON: But why does it happen?

FATHER: Well, it is a normal stage of development for boys. As you get older, you will become sexually aroused more often. You'll have sexual fantasies and thoughts, and sexual tension will build up in your body that needs to be released.

SON: But can't I take care of it with masturbation?

FATHER: That will help. But your body is going through incredible changes—hormones and all that. Sex will become so important to you that you're likely to have lots of sexual dreams and get aroused when you aren't awake to masturbate. As you get older and begin to have regular sexual outlets, the wet dreams will probably stop altogether.

Girls also need to know about nocturnal emissions, and boys need to know about menstruation, although not necessarily in as much detail. Once again, answer their questions without lecturing and without offering more than they can comprehend.

EXPLAINING ERECTIONS AND VAGINAL LUBRICATION

Again, both boys and girls need to know about erections and vaginal lubrication. You might explain these phenomena in the following way:

MOTHER OR FATHER: In order for intercourse to occur, three things have to happen. The first is that the male has to get an erection—his penis has to get hard. The penis gets erect when the male becomes sexually excited, when he feels warm and loving toward someone. When a female feels warm and loving and sexually excited, two things happen to her. Her body makes a fluid that is like a fine oil that lubricates the vagina. And the vagina actually opens up wider, wide enough so that the penis can fit inside it. It slides in easily because of the lubrication. This feels good for both the male and the female.

Explain that when a girl has sex for the first time, she may experience pain, and there may be some blood. This is because her hymen is broken. Also explain that just because there is no pain or blood, it does not mean that the girl is not a virgin. There are a number of ways that the hymen can be broken, including bicycle- and horseback-riding, gymnastics, and other physical activities.

If a girl's hymen is broken, and she is sufficiently relaxed and aroused to become lubricated, intercourse should not continue to be painful. If it is, your daughter may need to see a doctor. The doctor may either stretch her hymen or teach your daughter how to do so.

TALKING TO PRETEENS ABOUT AIDS

Most seventh- and eighth-graders are more comfortable learning about sexually transmitted disease and other sexual information at school in a formal academic setting than at home, which is usually more emotional and reserved as a safe place to revert to childhood. At school, in a classroom, sex is information, data, facts you must learn. At home there is always the innuendo that if you are interested or if you ask, it is because they "think you're doing something." Young teens are interested, and they do need to know, but they want to learn dispassionately, impersonally, in the abstract. They want and can handle the facts.

Research indicates that the majority of young people become sexually active with a partner before they leave their teens, and even if they do not, sexuality is a legitimate area of academic inquiry. Knowledge is always better than ignorance, and information about sex in general and STDs in particular will help them make better decisions about sexual activity. It is foolish, demeaning, and perhaps deadly to pretend that if they don't know about sex, they won't engage in it. It is a vote of confidence from parent to adolescent to be open about the inevitability and importance of sex in our lives and to provide information and counsel about sexual issues.

Discuss the topic of AIDS with your spouse/partner/adult friends casually in your household as you hear about it on the radio or TV or read about it in magazines and newspapers. Let your preteen overhear and contribute to these conversations. Give your child recognition for his or her knowledge on the subject. Ask if his or her friends worry about getting AIDS (most do not, because they do not see themselves at risk). Do not scare your preteen into a personalized fear of an AIDS death. If he or she has developed a personal fear of AIDS, reassure him or her about proper precautions, such as no drug use ever and safe-sex techniques when it's time to be sexual.

If you prepare your preteen for the myriad of changes that are going to occur to her or him physically and emotionally, you may save her or him a great deal of fear, anxiety, and embarrassment. In addition, by having frank, honest discussions about sex and by answering questions about sex in an open, nonjudgmental way, you may defuse some of your preteen's urge to experiment.

PARENTAL ISSUE: GOING BACK

Children who know their parents will not judge them, overreact, or preach will be more likely to ask questions. For this reason it is vital that parents have empathy for their children and understand what they are going through. Continue working on your own issues so that you can keep the lines of communication open.

Remember your preadolescent years, the sexual concerns you had, the fear and excitement you felt at the thought of sexual development. Did you have anyone to talk to about your concerns? Who told you about menstruation/nocturnal emissions? How was it explained to you? How did it make you feel about this inevitability? What attitudes were passed on to you about menstruation or nocturnal emissions? How did you feel about your body as it began to mature sexually? Were you an early bloomer or a late one?

For mothers, remember how you felt during the menarche—the beginning of menstruation. How did you feel about your breasts developing? About the growth of pubic hair? Perhaps you may want to share those feelings when you talk to your daughter about menstruation.

For fathers, remember the stage in your development marked by increased sensitivity to unexpected, unwanted, spontaneous erections, the beginning of masturbation and nocturnal emissions. Remember when you began to grow pubic hair, when your voice changed, sometimes in an embarrassing way. Were you proud or ashamed when these things happened? Were you teased by other family members or friends? Were you one of the slow starters in your circle of friends, or did you begin early and lead the others?

Despite the signs of maturation, children are still children at this age. Even though your child may experience sexual desire and may be capable of impregnating a girl or becoming pregnant, he or she is not emotionally equipped to have sex. The early teen is interested in exploring the possibilities of relationships and bonding, but there is much to learn before he or she is ready for sexual intercourse. Most early teens will tell you that they are just "not ready" for sex with a partner, without being able to explain why. Many are encouraged, goaded, seduced, or challenged into sexual behavior before it is in their best interest because adults have failed to provide enough information about sexual rights, responsibilities, and rewards for them to assert their right to decline. Some enter into sexual activities with peers or older partners in response to high levels of sexual interest, curiosity, and desire.

Studies show that children who are able to talk to their parents comfortably about sex and have a solid knowledge of their bodies and how they function postpone intercourse for a longer time than those who do not.

13

♦

Adolescence (Ages 13–18)

E ven though your child's attitudes about sexuality begin early based on parental messages and childhood experiences with sex, it is during puberty that her or his sexuality becomes the focus of her or his attention. Puberty is a time when the most profound physiological and psychological changes in our lifetime occur: the development of secondary sex characteristics, the acceleration of both physical and emotional growth, the capacity to reproduce, an increased involvement in both peer group and the other sex, the development of personal values, and the desire to behave more independently.

NORMAL STAGES OF PSYCHOSEXUAL DEVELOPMENT

Adolescence is a time for:

- ✦ Individuation
- ✦ "Fitting in"
- ✦ Dating and sexual decision-making
- ✦ Reexamining and sometimes rejecting their parents' values

✦ Searching for sexual identity
✦ Exploring, experimenting, and taking risks

ADOLESCENCE IS A TIME FOR INDIVIDUATION

Individuation, the act of a child becoming a separate "self" from his or her parents, is a major task of adolescence. To accomplish this, teenagers must gradually become more independent from their parents and take on more responsibility for themselves. This process often causes a certain amount of distancing between parent and child. But too much distancing can be harmful because teens still need their parents' support, acceptance, and guidance in order to move into adulthood.

The most important thing to keep in mind, as you deal with children of this age group, is that you probably will not know very much about their sexual thoughts and probably even less about their sexual behavior. Parents like to believe that their teen would consult them first if he or she were in need or in trouble. However, many adolescents report that their parents would be the last to know, because they would not be able to face them. Their need to be private and self-reliant is age-appropriate and a sign of strength, but it makes dealing with them about sexual matters difficult for most parents.

Your adolescent may try to convince you that she or he is not interested or that she or he already knows everything you are trying to explain. Your teen may listen to what you have to say, but offer nothing to sustain a dialogue for fear of revealing herself or himself. Your best attempts may sound like a lecture to your teen and end in your feeling frustrated and angry. It is important that you not become discouraged and remember your child still needs you, but in a slightly different way. Your teen depends on you to acknowledge and support his or her need to take increasing control over his or her own life, but to be there in the old ways when he or she is overwhelmed.

ADOLESCENCE IS A TIME FOR "FITTING IN"

For many young people, adolescence is one of the most difficult periods of life to get through. In addition to the confusion and anxiety about their physical development, there are pressures from all sides—to do well in school, to be popular, to compete scholastically, athletically, and socially, to plan for college, a career, and marriage, and somehow to come to terms with their sexuality. Questions like "Am I sexually attractive?" "What is my sexual orientation?" "Should I become sexually active?" plague most adolescents.

During adolescence, more than any other time in our lives, it is vitally important that we "fit in" with our peers. In addition to the pressures all teens feel, those who do not fit in with the crowd for one reason or another have a particularly difficult time.

This was the case with Marcus:

I was only five-foot-two-inches tall by the time I was sixteen years old. Being so short made me feel incredibly unattractive and inadequate. I was teased mercilessly and called names like "Shorty," "Midget," and "Pee Wee." I didn't dare ask a girl out because I just knew she would laugh at me, so instead I just acted like their pal. In fact, I was so insecure about my height that I didn't ask a woman out on a date until I was twenty years old, and that was only because she was shorter than I am and she came on to me first.

The need to belong becomes one of the most important issues in a teenager's life—so important that if he or she appears to be completely indifferent to group opinion, he or she is probably covering up feelings of isolation and estrangement, as was the case with Jess:

All during high school I convinced myself that I really didn't care whether I fit in or not. I developed a "screw-you" attitude and did the most outrageous things as a way of rebelling against all the group conformity bull. I held on to this attitude way into my twenties, until I finally realized that it was all a facade—I cared deeply what other people thought, especially women. It's just that I am so terribly insecure around them that it is painful.

For all these reasons and more, adolescence is a painful time for most teenagers. Because it is such a difficult stage, and because of all the changes going on inside their bodies, they are extremely sensitive, emotional, and changeable. They often feel like they are going to explode with emotions.

ADOLESCENCE IS A TIME FOR DATING AND SEXUAL DECISION MAKING

In the midst of all this upheaval, uncertainty, and worry, adolescents also have to deal with the issue of dating. For girls, the problem is whether or not anyone will ask them on dates or whether the *right* boys will ask them on dates. For boys, the issue is whether or not they can get up the courage to ask a girl out, and then of course, whether they can handle the humiliation if she says "no."

Each adolescent's attitude toward his or her physical and social competence, his or her body, his or her role as a male or female, and his or her new sexual feelings influences how he or she relates to the opposite sex. In addition, all of his or her earlier experiences with sexuality play a part in how the teenager feels about him or herself, and this in turn influences how he or she relates.

Once they get past the initial dating jitters, adolescents are then faced with another problem—what to do with their sexual feelings. The decision as to when to become sexually active is one that plagues not just girls but boys as well. The things that influence their decision are often religious beliefs, parental upbringing, and peer pressure. Often, these things are in conflict with one another, as they were with Todd:

I was raised in a very religious family, and I was taught that premarital sex is a sin. I had every intention of waiting until I was married to have sex, but I found that this decision was not an easy one to keep. I received a tremendous amount of pressure from the other boys to start having sex. They all talked about their sexual conquests and then would ask me about mine. At first I stood by my convictions and told them I wasn't going to have sex until I was married. But this soon gave me the reputation of being a nerd, or worse yet, a fag. I was taunted mercilessly by the boys, who began to call me "Virgin Mary."

Finally, to save face I lied about having sex with a girl I had been going out with. This got them off my back, but I felt terrible about lying about the girl. I was afraid that it would get back to her and she'd never speak to me again, and I really liked her a lot.

While some people choose to remain virgins, even into their thirties, most men and even most women become concerned if they are still virgins past the age of twenty-one. Things have changed even for females. Where remaining a virgin until a young woman's wedding night was once a virtue, today it has become a burden for many, as it is with Francesca:

I'm a twenty-three-year-old virgin, and I've reached a point where I'd just like to get it over with. I wish I had had sex a long time ago because now I've waited so long that it's become too big a deal. Now when a guy finds out I'm a virgin, he gets afraid. No one wants to be the first one. I've had guys tell me to come back after I've lost my virginity. But I don't want to lose it to just anyone either. I really feel trapped.

Some people choose to be virgins for religious reasons, believing that it is a sin to have sex before marriage. Others want to save themselves for that special person, as was the case with Michael, a twenty-eight-year-old virgin:

I just haven't met the right woman. It is really important to me that I be in love with the woman I have sex with, especially the first time. It's such a special experience, why waste it on someone you don't even care about?

And recently, there has been a new "chastity" movement among teenagers. Thousands of teens are making public commitments to remaining virgins until they get married.

ADOLESCENCE IS A TIME TO REEXAMINE AND SOMETIMES REJECT THEIR PARENTS' VALUES

During adolescence in particular, the values held by young people undergo examination and change. Young people enter adolescence with the values they have accumulated during their childhood—most often, those conveyed to them by their parents' words and actions. Usually these values have been accepted with little question. But in order for a young person to be able to act on these values, in order for them to become beliefs, especially when she or he is faced with the variety of freedoms and challenges the world offers, the adolescent must gain a different kind of "ownership" of these values. The adolescent must arrive at a point where the values are held because she or he personally believes in them, irrespective of whether or not the parent believes in them. This is all part of the individuation process.

This is an important process, but one that leaves the adolescent vulnerable. In order to get "ownership," the adolescent has to look at his or her childhood values through the filter of his or her expanding ideas and experiences. And he or she has to examine a bewildering variety of new values: those held by peers, those conveyed by the media, and those illustrated by public and private adult behaviors. Adolescents need temporarily to reject some family values and "try on" some of the new values, and in so doing they may even adopt new and different behaviors as a way of testing how the new values fit.

This can be an extremely difficult time for parents, as you may have already experienced. It may be reassuring to learn that research shows that most adolescents eventually choose a set of values quite similar to those with which they were raised.

ADOLESCENCE IS A TIME TO SEARCH FOR SEXUAL IDENTITY

Adolescence is a critical time because it is at this early age that young teens are making major lifestyle decisions. From now until about age nineteen, your teen will be trying on various identities in order to find the one that best suits her or him.

One of the major tasks of adolescence is to identify and come to accept one's sexual identity. Given the confusion caused by a teenager's developing body, hormonal imbalances, the attitudes of peers and society in general, not to mention religious teachings, it is no wonder that this is one of the most difficult of the developmental tasks.

For this reason it is vital that you provide your teenager with complete and accurate information about what it means to be a heterosexual, a homosexual, or a bisexual. You don't need to be concerned about this information causing your child to become homosexual or bisexual. Gender identity is fixed by this age, so there is little anyone can do to change it.

For example, while you are giving information about marriage and childbirth, keep in mind that your child may be lesbian or gay. By giving information about and showing acceptance for all sexual identities, you will be showing your child that you will accept her or him no matter what her or his sexual orientation ends up being. Research indicates that the true homosexual has no choice as to his or her sexual orientation.

Do not tolerate jokes in your home about homosexuality. Instead, give accurate, balanced information about homosexuality, bisexuality, and heterosexuality. Assure your teen that same-sex friendships are not the same as homosexual relationships, that having a homosexual experience does not make you gay or lesbian, that it is perfectly okay for teens to have "crushes" on teachers and others they admire of the same sex.

Inform your teen that it is also a false assumption that a person who has homosexual thoughts or dreams must be a homosexual. Mature people are aware that they have both homosexual and heterosexual feelings, even though most prefer sexual activities with members of the opposite sex. People who are afraid of their healthy sexual impulses have a problem no matter what their sexual orientation.

Let your teen know that it is not easy to judge a person's sexual orientation by appearance. Some "feminine"-looking men or "masculine"-looking women are heterosexual, and some "all-American" types are homosexual.

ADOLESCENCE IS A TIME TO EXPLORE, EXPERIMENT, AND TAKE RISKS

It is part of normal development for teens to experiment and take risks as they explore their sexuality. This is all part of the individuation process. Because teens take risks and experiment, be sure you discuss all possible issues surrounding sexual behavior well in advance of your teen's dating years. Teens should be given information on all the following:

✦ Dating etiquette
✦ Contraception
✦ Masturbation
✦ Pornography
✦ Teen pregnancy
✦ Date rape
✦ Sexually transmitted diseases
✦ AIDS
✦ Drug and alcohol abuse

In the "Areas for Discussion" section later in the chapter, there will be more on how to have these discussions and exactly what your teen needs to know about many of these subjects.

TALKING TO YOUR ADOLESCENT

You may think that you've taught your child basically everything he or she needs to know about sex at this point. But this is not true. Sexual development is an ongoing process, and so consequently, your work is far from over.

It is vitally important that during this stage you set aside specific times for sharing between yourself and your teenager.

This can be anytime that you can sit down in a relaxed way to exchange ideas and experiences.

Unfortunately, the only time many parents actually talk to their teenager is when they're complaining, criticizing, or explaining how to behave properly. This can lead to problems such as poor school performance, drug usage, and teenage pregnancies. Don't make the mistake of limiting your communication to trying to control your teen's behavior. Once serious behavior problems develop and all communication is directed toward discipline, a vicious cycle will develop. Balance discipline and structure with open communication. Encourage discussions in which your teenager shares feelings, hopes, and experiences. Through this kind of sharing, you'll be better able to understand what is happening in your teen's life and therefore be in a better position to guide and advise.

You can be as candid as you feel comfortable about your own adolescence. If you can share something about your sexual experiences, it might bring you and your child closer. But it is also all right to tell your child that you are not comfortable sharing the sexual part of your life with him or her. Your child can certainly understand that, since there will be many aspects of your child's own life he or she will choose not to share with you.

You will need to decide ahead of time whether you are comfortable talking with your teen openly or not. The more open, the better; but if you are not comfortable, tell your teen that although you *want* to talk openly, it is hard for you. Tell her or him you will do your best to answer any and all questions and that if you don't know something, you'll make sure to find out. Determine that you will take this opportunity to work on your embarrassment and work on your own sexual issues so you can be more open.

You may find that your teen is much more willing to sit down with you to discuss sex than ever before. Because he or she is experiencing new sensations and feelings, because he or she now has a personal stake in learning about sex, your child's interest will be heightened.

If, however, you have never talked about sex with your child before, you may find that now that you are approaching the subject, she or he absolutely refuses to talk with you about it. If this is your situation, begin the conversation something like this: "I can understand why you might feel embarrassed to talk with me now. I should have talked to you when you were younger." Plan ahead for such disclosures; have a book ready. Tell your teen that you think she or he might be interested in it. Explain that some of the material might embarrass her or him, but that you're going to leave the book around just the same. The main thing is for your child to understand that you are available to talk anytime she or he is ready. Another technique is to "hide" a book. Most teenagers are very adept at finding such "hidden" material.

Here are some of the most frequent concerns teenagers report having, things they are *not* likely to ask their parents:

✦ Am I masturbating too much?
✦ Do I have homosexual tendencies?
✦ Am I abnormal if I have thoughts about sex with people I know, even family members?
✦ Are my breasts too small? Too big?
✦ Is my penis too small? Too large?
✦ How can you tell if you have VD?
✦ Is there something wrong with me if I remain a virgin?
✦ How can I say "no"?
✦ How can I tell if I'm pregnant?
✦ Why do I have all these unexplained erections?

AREAS FOR DISCUSSION

✦ Setting rules and limits, including rules for dating
✦ Teaching sexual decision making
✦ Talking about contraceptives
✦ Talking about STDs
✦ AIDS and safe sex

+ Talking to your teen about homosexuality and homophobia
+ The "first time"
+ Talking about the latest sexual trends

SETTING RULES AND LIMITS, INCLUDING RULES FOR DATING

Although they will fight you all the way, teens actually feel more comfortable when they have clear limits and boundaries, when they know exactly what is expected of them. Teens need help learning strategies for coping with their sexual urges and drives. Setting reasonable boundaries on curfews, sleepovers, or parties is an important way to give your teen a sense of balance. It's easy for him or her to get out of control, and you can help bring him or her back to reality.

Many teens will be quick to tell you that nobody "dates" any longer, that they "hang out" or "go out." ("Hanging out" usually means a group of girls and boys getting together, not necessarily in matched pairs, but just as a "group" doing something together.) However, these situations aren't as loose or casual as teens try to make them sound. Almost all teens report that their initial attempt at a relationship with the opposite sex was planned just like a "date." The term "dating" still seems to be the best way to describe someone going out with the opposite sex by prior arrangement. Teens still use the word *date* and list concerns about "dating" when asked what they most want to talk about.

When?

There really is no pat answer to this question. Your son or daughter should gradually be allowed increasing independence and responsibility, and this includes dating. Most experts recommend a progression from adult-supervised group activities, to unchaperoned group activities that may include couples, to one-on-one experiences.

Determining when your teen is ready to go from one step to

another will depend on two things: maturity level and chrono-logical age (with maturity level being most important). Al-though it varies from family to family, there is a general agreement that teenagers under fourteen should only date in an adult-supervised manner and those over seventeen need not be chaperoned. In most communities, fifteen and sixteen are the most commonly acceptable ages to begin dating.

Experts have found that the best way to instigate dating rules is for the teen to be included in the process. It has been found that teens who are included in the rule-making process tend to be much better at following the rules. Otherwise, if you make the rules without their input, it will be an open invi-tation for rebellion.

Hear your teen out. Listen carefully to his or her point of view before you ultimately make your decision. Then don't set the rules in stone, but leave a little room for changes.

The following suggestions are meant as guidelines when es-tablishing dating rules in your household. They are based on both sound reasoning and the opinions of experts in the field.

1. *Know exactly where your teen is going on a date.* This is for her or his protection as well as your peace of mind.

2. *Set definite curfews.* As mentioned earlier, teens need limits. They promote structure and responsibility. Also, with-out a curfew, you have no way of knowing why your teen is not home yet—because he or she is in trouble or because he or she is just having a good time. You can give a later curfew as your son or daughter gets older and demonstrates the ability to handle responsibility.

3. *Insist on meeting all the boys your adolescent girl dates.* The boy who is willing to meet his date's parents is less likely to have something to hide than one who isn't willing to have this first meeting. Meeting parents will make him more likely to be motivated to act responsibly. Make sure the meeting is not interpreted as intimidation.

TEACHING SEXUAL DECISION MAKING

Children grow up faster these days and have to make decisions concerning their sexuality long before we ever did. Instead of trying to make your child's decisions for him or her, instead of "laying down the law" and insisting that he or she not have sex before age sixteen, or before eighteen, or before marriage, it will be far more effective if you continue to enhance your child's self-esteem by letting her or him know that you trust her or his judgment and by continuing to remind your child that her or his body is a wonderful gift and is worthy of respect and care.

Instead of panicking when your daughter begins to develop and becomes popular with the boys, instead of accusing your daughter of dressing like a "whore" or "slut," it is far more important that you stay in close contact with her, provide her with information, and guide her through the delicate choices she will be making.

Just what kind of information? Primarily information about responsibility. Teach your adolescent that it is his or her responsibility to select a girlfriend or boyfriend who is considerate, dependable, emotionally healthy, and respectful—someone who can make careful choices and respect another person's choices. (Refer back to Chapter Eight, "Teaching Sexual Values and Responsibility," for specific guidelines to offer your teen in terms of deciding whether a particular partner is a good choice for a sexual partner.)

And certainly you will want to remind your adolescent about sexual safety—including how to protect her or himself from unwanted pregnancies, that abortion is not synonymous with birth control, how to protect her or himself from sexually transmitted diseases, and what measures she or he can take to prevent rape (please refer to Part I for rape prevention information). We will discuss preventing pregnancy and STDs in later chapters.

Regardless of how much importance you place on virginity,

regardless of your religion's regard for chastity, most children will not postpone sex until marriage. (Seven out of ten young people are having sex before they are twenty-one.) Your child deserves to have the information he or she needs in order to make responsible choices.

By now your child is well aware of where you stand on sexual relationships at an early age and before marriage. Therefore, it makes no sense to *demand* that your child not have sex. If you are not sure he or she knows where you stand, then state your preference loud and clear, but do not scold or punish your child if he or she decides to become sexually active. The best you can do at this point is to make sure he or she continues with safety and responsibility.

There are several reasons why teenagers should be discouraged from having sex, and you should discuss these with your teen. For example, teenagers tend to be impulsive and for the most part (because of immaturity and inexperience) do not use good judgment. They do not have easy access to contraception, and teenage pregnancy is definitely unsound from medical and psychological points of view. (For example, the majority of teen mothers have premature babies.)

TALKING ABOUT CONTRACEPTION

It's never easy to acknowledge your child's sexuality, and talking to him or her about contraception is doing just that. It is acknowledging that there is a strong likelihood that your child will begin having sexual intercourse in the near future.

The other reason parents hesitate to talk to their adolescent about contraception is out of fear that they will then become promiscuous. Many of my clients have asked me through the years, "How can I talk to my teenage daughter about birth control without giving her the message that it's all right for her to have sexual intercourse?"

Many parents believe that teenagers equate information with consent, but this is not true. Your teenager knows very well what your values are. He or she knows how you feel about adolescent sex and premarital sex. If you like, you can preface the information you give with a statement reinforcing your values. You are giving information, not permission. It's one thing to tell a daughter that you will disown her if she becomes pregnant; it's quite another to explain your feelings something like this: "We really think you're too young to have intercourse, but if you're not going to listen to us, we urge you to practice birth control. We don't ever want you to feel that there's anything you can't talk to us about."

Many adolescents are under the false assumption that they can get away without using protection—"Just this once." Your teen needs to know that pregnancy can occur that one time and that an ovum can be fertilized even without intercourse. If the penis is on or near the labia when ejaculation occurs, sperm can make their way to the uterus. Even very small amounts of semen emitted prior to ejaculation can enter the vagina if the penis is in or near the vaginal area. Your teen also needs to know the advantages and disadvantages to the various methods of contraception and where to go for contraceptive materials. This does not mean that you have to be an authority on the various methods of preventing birth. Planned Parenthood has excellent material available, and many of the books listed in the Bibliography at the back of this book can also provide you with accurate information. While you can refer your child to these materials and books for information, you also need to explore the subject with your child because it is your guidance, interest, and concern that will help her or him make responsible choices.

Here is an example of the kind of discussion you might choose to have with your daughter:

MOTHER: I'd like to talk to you about contraception. This doesn't mean that your dad and I are giving you permission to go out and have sex. You know that we do not approve of sex for someone your age. But we also know that teens often get carried away, and so if you do decide to become sexually active, we want you to be responsible about it. That means protecting yourself from pregnancy and sexually transmitted diseases.

If you are going to be sexually active, you might want to consider the pill. It provides the most protection against pregnancy. You take a pill every day for three weeks and then stop for a week. A doctor has to prescribe the pill for you, and this means having a pelvic examination first. If you don't like the idea of taking chemicals, there are other choices, such as inserting vaginal foams, jellies, or sponges into the vagina just before intercourse. There is also the diaphragm, which is a rubber cap that fits over the cervix and prevents sperm from entering. The diaphragm needs to be fitted by a physician. It is fairly simple to insert, but it requires a bit of planning ahead if you're going to use it safely, and it must be used with a foam or jelly. When you use a diaphragm, jellies, or sponges, it is better if the man uses a condom to provide even more protection. The pill is safest and the most convenient, and it offers the best protection against pregnancy, but it will not protect you against sexually transmitted diseases.

While it is not 100 percent safe, a condom provides the best protection against both pregnancy and disease. The very best protection is using a condom in combination with a vaginal sponge or foam or diaphragm. You have to use a jelly with a condom anyway because without it you cause irritation to the tender tissue of your vagina.

You should also discuss responsibilities of sex in terms of love and kindness.

Boys need to receive a similar talk. This is the time when you come face-to-face with your values about sex—specifically, whether you feel boys should be "macho" and try sex as soon as possible or whether they should be more conservative, and how your son should treat females.

Your son needs to know that he has three choices every time he chooses to have sex: fatherhood, terminating life, or responsibility and precaution. He needs to know that if he gets a girl pregnant, he is equally responsible for the life of the baby. If the girl decides to keep the baby, he will be financially responsible for the child until it is eighteen years old. And if he thinks that abortion is the easy answer, he should know that more and more girls are choosing to keep their babies. Talk to him about the fact that an abortion is a serious business. He will be participating in terminating a life and responsible for at least half of the cost.

It doesn't matter if Mom or Dad does the talking, either together or separately. The most important thing to make clear to your adolescent is that if he or she chooses to become sexually active, *both* partners must be responsible for the prevention of pregnancy and disease.

TALKING ABOUT SEXUALLY TRANSMITTED DISEASES (STDs)

One out of five teens in the United States has been treated for a sexually transmitted disease. STDs include venereal diseases such as gonorrhea, syphilis, herpes, and the worst—AIDS. You don't have to become an expert on all STDs. Have some books on hand that explore STDs in greater depth than I am going to do here. It is helpful to have a quick source to refer to when you are talking with your teen. I have listed some in the Bibliography at the back of this book.

The following sexually transmitted diseases are listed with their possible symptoms, consequences, and available treatment.

CHLAMYDIA

SYMPTOMS IN WOMEN: Usually no symptoms; occasional vaginal discharge.

SYMPTOMS IN MEN: Usually discharge and painful urination.

WHEN SYMPTOMS APPEAR: 1–30 days after exposure.

SOME POTENTIAL CONSEQUENCES IF UNTREATED: Various inflammations, including pelvic inflammatory disease (PID) in women, which can lead to infertility and which increases the risk of ectopic pregnancy. A woman who is infected with chlamydia may pass it on to her infant during childbirth. (Adolescents have the highest rate of chlamydial infection, which is currently the most common of all STDs.)

TREATMENT: Broad-spectrum antibiotics (tetracycline). Recurrences possible.

GONORRHEA

SYMPTOMS IN WOMEN: Usually no symptoms; occasional vaginal discharge or painful, frequent urination, severe lower-abdominal or pelvic pain caused by PID (pelvic inflammatory disease).

SYMPTOMS IN MEN: Usually a yellow, thick discharge and severe burning sensation at the tip of the penis and pain when urinating. The penis becomes swollen and inflamed.

WHEN SYMPTOMS USUALLY APPEAR: *FOR WOMEN*: Specific symptoms may develop within two weeks or longer after exposure. *FOR MEN*: Usually within two to ten days after contact, but may remain without symptoms for a longer time.

POTENTIAL CONSEQUENCES IF UNTREATED: Various severe complications, including infertility in men and pelvic inflammatory disease in women, which can lead to sterility; will attack the joints and sex organs.

TREATMENT: Penicillin, related drugs (such as ampicillin), or other oral antibiotics. Strains that are more resistant require another round of same drug before patient is cured.

GENITAL WARTS

SYMPTOMS IN WOMEN: Single or multiple soft, fleshy growths around anus, vulva, vagina, or urethra. Usually painless, but can be uncomfortable.

SYMPTOMS IN MEN: Fleshy growths around anus or penis.

WHEN SYMPTOMS USUALLY APPEAR: One month to one year after exposure.

POTENTIAL CONSEQUENCES IF UNTREATED: These warts can be passed on to the infants of infected women during childbirth. Some studies show they may cause cervical cancer in women.

TREATMENT: Removal is the only treatment, but warts can grow back. If not removed by a doctor, they can multiply quickly.

HERPES

SYMPTOMS IN WOMEN: Single or multiple blisters or sores on or near the genitals. These may erupt and become small sores that may be painful, tender, or itchy. There may also be fever, headaches, or "flu-like" symptoms (feeling sick all over). The blisters are often very, very painful and may last up to three weeks. They disappear without scarring and may not surface again for some time. Whenever they do, the infected person may infect others.

SYMPTOMS IN MEN: Same as for women.

WHEN SYMPTOMS USUALLY APPEAR: 1–3 weeks after exposure.

POTENTIAL CONSEQUENCES: Cervical cancer believed to be more common in infected women. A mother who has herpes in the active stage may infect her infant during childbirth. More than half the infected infants die. Those who survive often have permanent brain damage.

TREATMENT: At this time there is no cure for herpes. However, a doctor can administer various ointments and oral tablets to reduce pain and itching and shorten duration of outbreak.

SYPHILIS

SYMPTOMS IN WOMEN: Four stages: 1) painless sore or chancre on the vagina, mouth, or rectum; 2) skin rash that does not itch or mucous patches, fever, sore throat, or aching body;

3) latent stage, no symptoms; 4) complications leading to possible death.

SYMPTOMS IN MEN: Same as for women except in first stage a painless sore forms on the penis, mouth, or rectum.

WHEN SYMPTOMS USUALLY APPEAR: 2–4 weeks after exposure.

POTENTIAL CONSEQUENCES IF UNTREATED: Death. Disease rarely progresses this far today. Adolescents who are sexually active and suffer from genital ulcers associated with syphilis or genital herpes are probably at greater risk of acquiring HIV. Several studies have shown that genital ulcers facilitate transmission of HIV.

TREATMENT: One to three massive doses (shots) of a special, long-acting type of penicillin brings the disease under control (complete cure).

AIDS (Acquired Immune Deficiency Syndrome)

SYMPTOMS IN WOMEN: After initial infection, a person may be asymptomatic for years. When an HIV-related illness progresses to symptomatic phase: fatigue, poor appetite, unexplained weight loss, persistent diarrhea, swollen glands, chronic dry cough, red or purple blotches on or under the skin (flat or raised), fever, chills, night sweats. In the last phase of AIDS, other infections cannot be resisted by damaged immune system.

SYMPTOMS IN MEN: Same as for women.

WHEN SYMPTOMS USUALLY APPEAR: May have no symptoms for years, but can still infect others.

POTENTIAL CONSEQUENCES IF UNTREATED: HIV infection progresses more rapidly to AIDS without treatment. Death.

TREATMENT: There is no cure for AIDS, although there are some medicines and treatments that can slow down the virus.

In general, a female should seek medical treatment for STDs if she has any of the following symptoms: a burning sensation while urinating; pain or itchiness in or around the vagina; a persistent sore throat; any soreness or redness around the vulva or anus; any sores or warts in or near the vulva; a discharge that is yellow, green, or discolored (a normal discharge is usually clear or milky); a thick discharge that looks like cottage cheese.

Generally speaking, a male should seek medical treatment if he has any of the following symptoms: a persistent sore throat; burning during and shortly after urination; any sores or warts on the penis or around it; any unusual coloring of the urine, such as urine that is reddish or very dark; a milky or puslike discharge; any soreness or redness around the anus.

Stress to your daughter or son that immediate treatment is crucial if she or he contracts an STD. Your child will be more likely to seek treatment if you stress that contracting an STD is nothing to be ashamed of and can happen to anyone. Make your teenager aware of community resources so that he or she can seek help on his or her own in case he or she is too embarrassed to confide in you. (Please note: Bacterial infections can cause many of the same symptoms as STDs. Reassure your teen that you will not assume they are sexually active if they complain of symptoms similar to those listed above.)

WHAT YOUR TEEN NEEDS TO KNOW ABOUT AIDS AND SAFE SEX

Older teens need to know that they are in particular danger of contracting AIDS. This is true for many reasons:

✦ No matter how afraid they are of contracting AIDS, their natural sexual interest, curiosity, and desire are extremely high, and their sexual drive is strong and demanding. Therefore, they may be driven to take more risks than an adult might.

✦ Spontaneous sexual encounters may find them unprepared to protect themselves from pregnancy and STDs.

✦ Sexual experimentation with more than one partner is common in mid-to-late teens.

+ Many teens are also experimenting with drugs.
+ Inexperience, lack of knowledge, and embarrassment make it difficult to negotiate for safe-sex practices.
+ Teens (especially girls) are reluctant to buy, carry, and use condoms.
+ Many girls use no protection at all against pregnancy or STDs.
+ Many girls have sex for nonsexual reasons and do whatever the boy wants because they want the boy.
+ Girls who have sex with older men might choose partners who are in high-risk groups.
+ Girls might have sex with boys who are having sex with other boys/men or prostitutes.
+ Boys might have sex with other boys/men or prostitutes.
+ Homosexual or bisexual boys might have high-risk sexual activity with partners in high-risk groups.
+ Most teens have few or no resources for accurate information about sexual matters and counsel.
+ Teens are reluctant to talk to any adult about their sexual activity.
+ Most teens have not been taught how to put on a condom or warned never to use a condom that has been carried around for a long time.

Seventy-five thousand American teens have contracted AIDS. While every teen is at risk of contracting AIDS, some are more at risk than others. Teach your teen how to determine his or her level of risk by sharing the following information:

+ Understand that HIV is transmitted sexually by exchanging body fluids with an infected partner. It is also transmitted by sharing intravenous drug needles with an infected person.
+ It is highly unlikely that you will know if your partner has been exposed to the virus. That person might not even know.
+ The more partners you have, the greater possibility you have of exposure to AIDS and other STDs.

+ Familiarize yourself with the high-risk groups (gay or bisexual men, intravenous drug users, prostitutes and their customers). If you are in a high-risk category or decide to have sex with someone who is, you will need to take precautions by using a condom, not sharing needles, and making sure there is no exchange of bodily fluids (blood, semen, or vaginal fluid).

+ If you have unsafe sex with a prostitute or with a male who has sex with prostitutes, you increase your risk of exposure.

Whether your teen feels at risk or not, whether he or she has made a commitment to chastity or not, he or she needs to know how to practice safe sex. He or she needs to know more than the fact that he or she should use condoms. Your teen needs to know the following:

+ Barriers that prevent the exchange of body fluids are your best line of defense and the use of spermicides make them even safer.

+ He or she should buy and use condoms lubricated with nonoxynol-9.

+ You can purchase condoms in any drugstore, no questions asked.

+ If a girl gives a boy the choice of sex with a condom and no sex without a condom, he will choose sex. (The choices should never include sex without a condom.)

+ You should never have sex when drunk or high, because you will tend to be more careless about using precautions.

+ Don't be talked into unprotected sex because neither of you has condoms or because the boy says it isn't natural, doesn't feel as good, he won't love you anymore, he'll find someone else, or any other excuse.

+ Don't be talked into sex for nonsexual reasons. Don't believe that if you give sex because your partner wants it, he or she will like you better or longer. They might just like sex and are willing to say anything to convince you to have it.

+ Don't depend on your partner to provide protection or good judgment in all sexual situations. He or she may put pressure on you when drunk or high or particularly horny. You need the courage to stand firm even if you are begged or threatened.

✦ Don't share intravenous drug needles, and don't have unprotected sex with anyone who does or has in the past shared drug needles.

✦ Most of the sexual activities called petting, including mutual masturbation to climax, are safe (and satisfying).

✦ Sexual orientation has no relationship to one's risk for AIDS. The risk of contracting HIV is related solely to coming into contact with the virus. This means taking part in unsafe sex practices with someone who is already infected. It does not matter if these are with men or women, gay or straight or bisexual. What does matter is practicing safe sex.

✦ The desire, urgency, and pleasure of the moment are not worth the risk of unprotected sexual intercourse.

✦ Many young people reserve sexual intercourse for marriage or a committed relationship.

SAFE SEX GUIDELINES

The following guidelines are recommended by The Institute for Advanced Study of Human Sexuality in *The Complete Guide to Safe Sex:*

Safe or Very Low Risk

✦ Sexual fantasies
✦ Sex talk (romantic, simply informational, or "talking dirty")
✦ Flirting
✦ Hugging
✦ Social (dry) kissing
✦ Phone sex
✦ Bathing together (including erotic bathing)
✦ Body massage (including erotic and nongenital oral massage)
✦ Smelling bodies and body fluids

+ Tasting our own body fluids
+ Body licking (on healthy, clean skin versus skin that has cuts, sores, or open wounds)
+ Consensual exhibitionism and voyeurism (showing off and watching)
+ Masturbation (mutual or solitary—penile, vaginal, clitoral)
+ Using personal sex toys
+ S&M games (without bruising or bleeding)
+ Sensuous feeding
+ Sex movies, videos, and tapes
+ Erotic books and magazines
+ Live sexual entertainment

Probably Safe, Possibly Risky

+ French kissing
+ Fellatio without ejaculation (safer with a condom)
+ Fellatio with ejaculation while wearing a condom
+ Cunnilingus (oral-vaginal sex, safer with a latex barrier and/or spermicide)
+ Peno-vaginal intercourse with condom (safer with spermicide, safer yet when combined with a cervical barrier—diaphragm, cap, or sponge)
+ Digital-anal sex with glove
+ Anal intercourse with condom (safer to withdraw before ejaculation)
+ Anilingus with latex (anal-oral sex, rimming through a rubber dam or condom)
+ Contact with urine

Unsafe

+ Vaginal intercourse without a condom
+ Anal intercourse without a condom
+ Swallowing semen
+ Receiving semen vaginally
+ Unprotected oral-anal contact

✦ Unprotected manual-anal intercourse
✦ Unprotected manual-vaginal intercourse
✦ Sharing menstrual blood
✦ Sharing needles or blood while piercing or shooting drugs

Some Poor Strategies

The following have been suggested in the past as risk-reduction strategies, but are *not recommended* anymore:

Be monogamous. This is a setup for someone to lie to you. If you believe your partner is monogamous and he or she is not, then you are being unknowingly exposed. If your partner is unfaithful, he or she may be afraid to tell you for fear of your leaving or not trusting him or her in the future.

A negative antibody test means it is safe. There are still false negatives (test says you are not infected, when in fact you are) and false positives (test says you are infected, but you are not). Also, an HIV infection can take several months to produce the antibodies that make the test results turn positive, and you may still be infectious during that time. And last but not least, you may have contracted the virus since you took the test.

Reduce your number of sex partners. Reducing the number of partners does reduce the risk of coming in contact with an infected partner, but it really depends on your choice of sex partners. It only takes one partner to infect you.

Be abstinent. This strategy is one way of stopping the transmission of AIDS, but it does not work for everyone. Suppressing sexuality is virtually an impossibility for most people, and it doesn't make sex go away. Some people who abstain from sex for a period of time often go on sexual binges in which they are totally unprepared to practice safe sex and wind up engaging in extremely risky activities. This then causes feelings of extreme fear and guilt followed by abstinence, and the cycle continues.

If your teen is reluctant to talk to you about this subject, suggest that he or she find a knowledgeable adult with whom he or she can discuss personal sexual concerns, someone the teen trusts enough to tell everything. There are sex information hotlines in most cities. Look in your directory for the number and give it to your teen. Tell your child that if she or he needs personal information and wishes to remain anonymous, she or he can call that number. If you have no sex information hotline in your area, see if there is an AIDS Foundation Hotline; or check your local gay community service center for a hotline. Please refer to Appendix I for addresses and phone numbers.

TALKING TO YOUR TEEN ABOUT HOMOSEXUALITY AND HOMOPHOBIA

Don't assume that just because your daughter or son has not brought up the subject of homosexuality that she or he is not interested in the subject. Teens are curious about what exactly homosexuality is, how you can tell if someone is homosexual, and what "causes" it.

Most teens believe that homosexuality is a very negative thing. In fact, homophobia—fear and hostility toward homosexuality—is rampant among adolescents. In addition, traditional scriptural prohibitions condemning homosexuality influence our culture to such an extent that it is not surprising many people are intolerant of homosexuality. For these reasons, teens are unlikely to bring up the subject with their parents.

Many teens fear that if they show an interest in the subject, they will arouse suspicions about their own sexual orientation, particularly if they are not involved with someone of the opposite sex, if they are having homosexual dreams or fantasies, or if they have a crush on someone of the same sex. Any of these situations can cause your teen to fear that he or she is homosexual.

The most important reason for bringing up the subject with your teen is the possibility that your son or daughter is either beginning to suspect or to become aware that his or her sexual preference is in fact for partners of the same sex. If you show your child that you are open and understanding about the subject, he or she will be more likely to confide in you. In the next chapter we will discuss how to handle it if your teen does feel he or she is homosexual.

Even if it is not a personal issue for your teen, it is important for her or him to be informed about the subject. Your teen may have friends, classmates, relatives, or acquaintances who are gay or lesbian. Being informed about the subject will help your child to handle not only her or his own fear and hostility, but the homophobia of others.

Although homophobia cannot prevent homosexuality, it discourages females from being assertive and males from being sensitive. Since conformity is celebrated among teens, even minor eccentricities bring on horrible teasing and even ostracism. If your child exhibits even the slightest deviation from stereotypical "masculine" or "feminine" behavior or fashion, he or she is fair game to be called queer, faggot, fairy, or dyke.

Initiate the discussion by using a TV program, book, or magazine article. Be as factual as you can and try to remain calm if he or she makes homophobic comments or jokes. Your teen is just parroting the anti-gay sentiments of his or her peers.

Begin by explaining to your teen that homosexuality is not abnormal; it is similar to being left-handed in a world of mostly right-handed people. And although there are many theories, no one really knows what causes homosexuality. There is abundant evidence, however, that homosexuality is not a choice, but a deeply felt, compelling orientation.

Most therapists and researchers agree that heterosexual and homosexual orientation are not distinct entities, but points on a continuum. The following scale of possible sexual behaviors was devised by Alfred Kinsey and his colleagues:

0: Exclusively heterosexual behavior
1: Largely heterosexual but incidental homosexual behavior
2: Largely heterosexual but more than incidental homosexual
    behavior
3: Equal amounts of heterosexual and homosexual behavior
4: Largely homosexual but more than incidental heterosexual
    behavior
5: Largely homosexual but incidental heterosexual behavior
6: Exclusively homosexual behavior

There are an estimated twenty million adults in the United States who are predominantly homosexual in their sexual and affectional orientation. This widely accepted estimate is supported by statistics provided in 1977 by the Kinsey Institute for Sex Research: 13.95 percent of males and 4.25 percent of females—or a combined average of 9.13 percent of the total population—had either extensive or more than incidental homosexual experience.

Thirty-seven percent of the white male population had at least one homosexual experience that led to orgasm. As for females, Kinsey suggested that, by age forty, 19 percent had had an erotic experience with another woman or women, but only about 2 to 3 percent were mostly or exclusively homosexual all their lives.

One of the most interesting things that Kinsey brought to our attention was that we cannot divide human sexuality into two categories called "heterosexuality" and "homosexuality." People are capable of both kinds of responses to varying degrees at different times in their lives. Sooner or later one sexual orientation usually dominates, but how or why this happens is not clear.

Not only do most of us fall somewhere on the continuum between heterosexuality and homosexuality, but our rating on the scale can change over time. The Kinsey people warn that their scale should not be seen as a series of rigid, fixed descriptions that necessarily describe all behaviors or predict future behaviors, because it has become clear that people do not necessarily maintain the same sexual orientation throughout their lives. Some people have a consistent homosexual orientation for a long period of time, then fall in love with a person of the opposite sex; other individuals who have had only opposite-sex partners later fall in love with a same-sex partner. And these changes are not usually a matter of "choice," just as a person can't will or force himself or herself to "fall in love" with some particular person.

There are several factors that determine your sexual orientation, including:

1. How you feel inside
2. How you identify yourself
3. Whom you choose to be with sexually

Teens also want to know about bisexuality, or as they often call it, "AC/DC" or "switch-hitting." Bisexuals are those who have sex with either male or female partners. Bisexuality seems to prove out Kinsey's continuum theory.

Others strongly believe that bisexuality is not a combination of heterosexuality and homosexuality; rather it is an entity by itself, a complete and distinct sexual orientation, where erotic attraction to both sexes is present.

There are many "straight" men who occasionally have sex with men, a number of gay men who periodically have sex with women, and most lesbians have related sexually to men at some point in their lives. Some straight women are occasionally attracted to other women. Bisexual people may have desires and fantasies for both sexes, but might relate only to one or the other.

Therefore, someone's statement that he or she is heterosexual, homosexual, or bisexual may not accurately indicate the extent of his or her sexual activities.

It is very important that you stress to your teen that sexual experiences with someone of the same sex does not mean the person is homosexual, and it does not *make* your teen homosexual. Most people have had sexual experiences with someone of the same sex during their childhood or adolescence.

Adolescents in particular tend to do a lot of exploring, including same-sex experiences. Convey to your teen that this kind of experimentation and having attractions to the same sex are all a normal part of growing up.

Girls seem to be less troubled by their same-sex experiences than boys. There is more permission in society for girls to hold hands, to hug, and to be together all the time. It is even more acceptable for girls to go through a stage of having a deep crush on another girl, and even if sex play takes place, neither girl tends to see herself as a lesbian. Typically, as their relationships with boys increase, their crushes on girls decrease, but some girls worry that their feelings or experiences are not normal.

Your son or daughter may ask you how a person knows if he or she is gay or lesbian. Many of my homosexual clients report that they suspected they were gay or lesbian even before they had actual sexual experiences with someone of the same sex. They remember always feeling uncomfortable or emotionally empty when they were with opposite-sex partners, but very comfortable and satisfied with a same-sex partner. Some of my homosexual clients say they went through a slow process of discovering that they were gay or lesbian. And still others experienced a long struggle trying to fit in as a heterosexual and discovering that they just weren't being true to themselves. Many people do not discover that they are primarily attracted to and sexually compatible with others of the same sex until they are adults, maybe not until they have been married and have children. (Most of the research indicates that self-discovery of homosexuality is most likely to occur during adolescence for males and a somewhat later time for females. A large number of lesbians do not adopt homosexuality until after a heterosexual marriage.)

However, adolescence is the primary time when gay males and lesbian females first become aware that they are not sexually attracted to the opposite sex. This, of course, makes them feel different and alone. Most keep their feelings hidden from family and friends and are terrified of being "found out" before they are willing to tell. While heterosexual teenagers are learning about dating and establishing relationships, gay teens are not learning any of that; they are learning instead to hide their feelings. Lesbian girls are usually more isolated than gay boys. They have fewer resources for meeting other young lesbians. Because of all the secrecy and fear, you will need to be alert to any signals your son or daughter may be sending you.

TALKING TO YOUR TEEN ABOUT "THE FIRST TIME"

The clumsy initial intimacies of adolescence may have an excitement that will never again be matched throughout life. On the other hand, this very clumsiness can be devastating. Lack of accurate information about sex may shape our first sexual experiences with another person, and that experience—good or bad—often colors our general feelings about sex.

Our first sexual experience with another person can set the tone for our sexuality. If it is basically positive—with tenderness, mutual respect, and caring, then we are not so devastated by later negative sexual experiences. But if our first sexual experience with another person is painful or humiliating, we are far more likely to believe that sex is a negative experience.

Our first sexual experience is highly charged. The sights, sounds, smells, and sensations of that first experience often remain indelibly imprinted in our mind and in our body. Whether the experience was a good one or a bad one, whether it was by choice or by force or coercion, the fact remains that the experience was extremely powerful and stimulating. Because of this, we will often replay that first experience over and over in our lifetime, whether it is reflected by our choice of partner or our preference in terms of location, position, or type of sexual act.

Our first sexual experience can either be a wonderful experience, opening us up to our passions and the pleasure of intimacy, or it can sour us on the idea of sex. It can be fulfilling or embarrassing, something to "get over" or something to savor, something that whets our appetite for more or something that turns us off.

For these reasons, your teen needs to know what to expect "the first time." Warn your teen that his or her first forays into sex may not always be enjoyable. Because they are nervous and inexperienced, boys often become so excited that they ejaculate prematurely. Because it is over in such a short amount of time and because they are nervous, girls seldom experience an orgasm and may often experience pain if their hymen is still in place.

Suggest that if your teen is going to have sex (again, this does not mean you are giving your approval), she or he chooses a place that feels safe and where she or he can be relaxed and unhurried.

TALKING TO YOUR TEENAGER ABOUT THE LATEST SEXUAL TRENDS

In addition to discussing the typical struggles of adolescence, you also need to talk to your teen about current sexual trends. As we discussed earlier, teens will experiment and take risks in their attempt to individuate and discover their true sexual nature. And since teens are overly concerned about "fitting in" with their peers, they are particularly vulnerable to getting caught up in sexual trends that may be damaging.

Those who are young and impressionable are often introduced to types of sexuality that they wouldn't have thought about or become interested in on their own. These activities may at first seem exciting, and their natural curiosity may get the better of them, or they may go along with activities in order to be accepted or in order to hold on to a sexual partner.

Parents today cannot afford to be prudish or squeamish when it comes to sex. Primarily due to the fear of AIDS, many sexual practices that were once considered "fringe" or "kinky" are now openly discussed and acted out in the general public. Your teenager is going to hear about these practices from peers, from television talk shows, videos, films, and newspapers, so you had better educate yourself about them as well. Below I have listed some of the most popular sexual trends that are catching on with adolescents.

Phone Sex

Like it or not, your teenager will probably at one time or another experience curiosity about phone sex. Because he or she is bombarded with phone sex advertisements on television, particularly late at night when teens tend to watch MTV and some of the other cable stations that cater to teens, it is a rare teen who will not succumb to the temptation. You may have already discovered this due to an outrageous phone bill or two, or you may have accidentally walked in on your teen while he or she was in the middle of such a conversation. You can put a block on your telephone to prevent anyone in your household from making such calls, but that won't necessarily prevent your teen from making the calls. He or she can still call from a friend's house or set up his or her own (noncommercial) phone sex line with friends.

Phone sex has become very popular and is as widespread as it is today primarily because of AIDS. Some people, especially those involved in AIDS prevention, advocate phone sex as an excellent alternative to more dangerous forms of sex, especially among young people. They believe that the popularity of phone sex confirms what sexologists have said all along—that sex is more about what is happening between our ears than what is going on between our legs.

We all know what commercial phone sex is all about, but what about noncommercial phone sex? What is it exactly? Phone sex commonly refers to consensual behavior (not to be confused with illegal, nonconsensual, harassing, and obscene phone masturbation calls) such as listening to a lover or friend talk in a provocative, sexy voice on the other end of the telephone.

Phone sex includes:

✦ Reading erotic literature to your partner over the phone
✦ Telling your partner, in graphic detail, what you'd like to do to them if you could
✦ Pretending to be strangers

+ Asking how your partner is dressed or undressed
+ Telling each other about previous sexual experiences

You cannot control your teen at all times, particularly if she or he has a phone in her or his room. If you suspect (or know) that your teen is involved in phone sex, instruct her or him to get consent from anyone she or he would like to call and to negotiate the parameters of these calls. (Is it okay to call late at night? Are there some words, fantasies, or suggestions that would be upsetting to you?) Make certain that your teen understands that talking sexual to people on the phone when there is no prior agreement is considered an obscene phone call and that obscene phone calls are illegal and can be traumatic to the person who is forced to listen.

Even though you may disapprove of phone sex, whether commercial or noncommercial, it is a popular fad and one that your teen will likely experiment with. The best you can hope for is that your teen satisfies his or her curiosity quickly and does not get "hooked" on it (particularly commercial phone sex, which can be expensive).

Voyeurism

Voyeurism is the fastest-growing form of sex, and it is considered the safest form of sex in the age of AIDS. It includes watching pornographic movies, watching someone undress, watching other couples make love, and watching strippers (recent studies show that there has been a 50 percent increase in the number of strip clubs in the country).

But voyeurism has also taken a more dangerous turn. More and more, males are spying on girls in order to see them undress or make love with another male. This is not the same as young boys sneaking a look into the girls' dormitory. Many young men today are becoming obsessive about watching young women, and when the girls find out about it, they feel victimized, enraged, and humiliated.

Some young men go so far as to work together in order to

videotape sex sessions with girls. A young man takes a girl to his apartment and has sex with her, and all the while his buddy is hiding in the closet videotaping the entire scene. The two men then view the tapes later on. Some of the young men show the tapes to all their friends, and some have even sold the tapes.

Many voyeuristic acts are against the law. While teens and young people may think it is exciting and fun, it is nevertheless an invasion of privacy and can cause emotional damage to those whose privacy they are invading. It can also lead to public humiliation (if not arrest) to those who do it, as it did in Zack's case:

> I started peeping in my neighbors' windows when I was fifteen. I'd heard other guys talk about it, and it was exciting to see half-naked and naked women parading around the house. But after a couple of months a neighbor set a trap for me, and I got caught. He had tied a rope across his yard, which happened to be the path I used to get to some of the houses where I peeped. I felt so humiliated when he came running out, and I felt even worse when two neighbors pressed charges against me.

Educate your teen about the various forms of voyeurism, those that are relatively harmless as well as those that are more invasive and damaging. Make certain that he or she understands the difference between consensual voyeurism (such as "pretending" to catch someone undressing or masturbating) and actually sneaking around and invading someone's privacy.

Exhibitionism

Exhibitionism, like voyeurism, is at an all-time high, again probably because of AIDS. Some argue that it reduces the risk factor both sexually and emotionally.

A true exhibitionist is someone who becomes sexually aroused by exposing his or her naked body or genitals to others or performing sexual acts in front of others. But young people are also becoming involved in exhibitionism as a trend. Many young people are exposing themselves in public places just for fun and for the shock value. Needless to say, this kind of activity can expose both young women and young men to rape.

Believe it or not, more and more young women are deciding to become professional strippers. They argue that it is "old-fashioned" to think of strippers as being exploited—that in fact, strippers have a great deal of power over men. Many college students (male and female) work as strippers as a way of earning extra money, and some do it to pay their way through college. In addition, many young people who aspire to be professional dancers or actors often think that stripping is a good way to be "discovered."

Make certain that your teen has not "romanticized" the idea of stripping—give her or him the facts. Stripping can be extremely degrading and can expose your child to a subculture of drugs and prostitution. It often turns young people off sex because it exposes them to a very seedy population of people. Seldom does a young person get "discovered" as a stripper unless it is for pornographic films.

Bisexuality

Another type of sexual behavior that has become increasingly popular among teens is bisexuality. Some teens have become drawn to this behavior because their favorite rock, punk, or pop star is bisexual or dresses and acts as if they are (Prince, Madonna, Michael Stipe of R.E.M.). Others may experiment with it just because their friends are into it, while still others may be doing it to get a rise out of their parents or to get attention. And some may truly be discovering their sexual orientation.

If your teen believes he or she is truly bisexual, you will need to educate yourself and your child about this sexual orientation (refer to previous discussion). While bisexuality may be trendy, true bisexuals are often criticized and ostracized by both heterosexuals and homosexuals. Homosexuals accuse them of not being willing to risk coming out of the closet, while heterosexuals accuse them of being unwilling to make a choice and "having their cake and eating it too." Individuals in both groups shy away from them because they see them as confused and not able to be monogamous.

If your teen is experimenting, make sure he or she understands that you can have same-sex experiences without being either homosexual or bisexual and that there is plenty of time to discover his or her true sexual orientation.

Sadomasochism (S&M)

Sadomasochism refers to the consensual eroticizing of power or the exploration of intense tactile sensation. S&M is a type of sexual activity that was once confined to only a small portion of our population. Today, celebrities like Madonna have brought this practice into the limelight and made it popular with a much larger segment of people, most notably young people in their teens and twenties, gays and lesbians, and those in the avant-garde.

Madonna's video for the song "Human Nature" shows her dressed in black leather along with whips and chains, actively involved in sadomasochistic activities. Her message in the song is, "Express yourself, don't repress yourself." Many believe it is irresponsible of Madonna, whose majority of fans tend to be ten-to-thirteen-year-old kids, to be advocating S&M.

Whatever your personal feelings are about sadomasochism, it is important to realize that teenagers are not emotionally equipped to handle such a sexual activity. Sexuality is overwhelming enough for young people without having to deal with the complex issues of pairing sex with power, submission, and physical pain.

Until recently, researchers had estimated that 5 to 10 percent of the U.S. population engaged in sadomasochism for sexual pleasure on at least an occasional basis, with most incidents being either mild or staged activities involving no real pain or violence.

It appears that many more individuals prefer to play the masochist's role than the sadist's. It also appears that males are more likely to prefer sadomasochistic activities than females. This means that male sadomasochists may have difficulty in finding willing females to be sexual partners.

If partners are located, an agreement is reached about what will occur. The giving and receiving of actual or pretended physical pain or psychological humiliation occurs in most cases only within a carefully prearranged script. Any change from the expected scenario generally reduces sexual pleasure.

Most often it is the receiver (the masochist), not the giver (the sadist), who sets and controls the exact type and extent of the couple's activities. In many such heterosexual relationships, the so-called traditional sex roles are reversed—with men playing the submissive or masochistic role.

There are many young people who are talked into S&M and who get in over their heads before they know what is happening, as was the situation with Laurie:

> When I was just seventeen, an older boyfriend that I was madly in love with introduced me to sadomasochism. The whole idea of it scared me, and he had to do a lot of persuading to get me involved, but he gradually got me over my fears, and I tried it. We started out doing some really mild things, like having him tie me up and blindfold me. This was kind of exciting since I could fantasize that he was forcing me and not have to feel guilty about having sex like I sometimes did. But gradually, things kind of got out of control. He started hitting me with a whip while I was tied up and putting clips on my nipples.
>
> You have to understand that I was really crazy about this guy, and he was really an exciting guy to be around. He had lots of interesting friends, and we were always going to these really neat parties and sometimes even meeting celebrities. A lot of his friends were into the same kind of thing, so it seemed almost normal at the time.
>
> When he started to get rougher with me and actually hurt me, I tried to tell him that I really didn't like it. But I wasn't

very forceful about it, and he was very persuasive, telling me all about the fact that I was increasing my ability to experience sexual pleasure and what an exciting lover I was and how he didn't need anyone but me. And so I let it go on, even though I was sometimes really frightened and was often physically hurt.

After a while, the experience started taking its toll on me though, not only physically, but emotionally. I started to dislike myself for letting my boyfriend treat me as he did and for not standing up to him. And he started treating me like a slave or a whore outside of the bedroom as well. He'd order me around and expect me to do whatever he wanted. Gradually, I stopped hanging out with my friends because I knew they wouldn't understand what I was into. I felt ashamed of myself when I was around my family, so I stopped seeing them very often too. I became more and more isolated, until I only associated with my boyfriend and his friends.

As I became more and more dependent on my boyfriend, he became more and more abusive to me in and out of bed. I wanted to leave him, but I didn't feel strong enough. Eventually, he left me for another woman. It has taken me three whole years to recover from that relationship and to be able to hold my head up with people and not feel horribly ashamed.

Warn your teen that even though sadomasochism is trendy, it can be dangerous. Let him or her know that sex is complicated enough at that age without complicating it further by involving power, submission, and pain-as-pleasure.

Body Piercing

Piercing the ears has been acceptable for women for centuries and has even become popular with men in the past twenty years or so. Among the punk chic, multiple ear piercing is the fashion for both sexes. Those who engage in piercing as an erotic form of sexual expression claim that there is greater sensitivity to the nipple, labia, or penis once it is pierced. Sometimes it is also an act of submission in a mutual and consensual exchange of power (sadomasochism).

Piercing presents some concerns. When the skin is free of nicks, cuts, or open sores, there is no necessity to worry about any blood, semen, vaginal juices, urine, or feces that might be deposited on it. Depending on how long a person's body takes to heal after a piercing, it is possible for any of these fluids to enter the body and transmit the HIV virus.

But the more serious problem is similar to that of sharing needles in intravenous drug use. If your teen is into piercing, make sure he or she uses sterilized equipment and never shares it. The supplies involved are inexpensive and readily available, so everyone should have his or her own set. Frequently, in large cities, tattoo or piercing parlors will perform the piercing safely. Get the names of professional piercers who are AIDS aware (who use single-use needles, wear gloves, and keep their equipment sterilized). Probably the safest way to have it done is to ask your physician to do it.

Water Sports

"Water sports" or "golden showers" refer to urinating on or in someone. This practice may sound bizarre to you, but it is an integral part of some sexual lifestyles such as S&M. You should at least be aware of its existence, and if you discover that your teen is involved in this, warn your child that he or she can contract AIDS if the person urinating on him or her is HIV-positive. There are precautions he or she can take, such as wearing a latex body suit.

Don't make the mistake of thinking that your teen would never get involved with these "fringe" or "kinky" practices. Because these practices are so "trendy," more and more young people are experimenting with them.

The purpose of my listing these popular sexual trends is not to scare you, but to make you aware of their existence so you can pass on the information to your child. Teens often get talked into these kinds of activities without really understanding the dangers. If you can educate your child about these dangers ahead of time, you may save her or him a lot of needless pain.

In addition, adolescents and young people often get involved with sexual practices that can lower their self-esteem. An esteem-robbing sexual practice is any sexual activity that causes us to feel bad about ourselves, either because the act is something that goes against our values and belief system, or because the act itself is emotionally (or even physically) damaging to us.

Sex should make us feel attractive, stimulated, excited, sensuous, and ultimately, relaxed and appreciated—if not loved (often in this order). In short, it should make us feel good about ourselves. Esteem-robbing sex may make us feel many of the same things initially, but ultimately, we end up feeling remorse, shame, guilt, and humiliation.

Unfortunately, esteem-robbing sex can become addictive, and young people find that they continue the behavior even against their better judgment. Time after time they repeat the behavior, and time after time they promise themselves they will stop. A vicious cycle is created: The more they engage in the negative behavior, the worse they feel about themselves; and the worse they feel about themselves, the more they engage in the behavior.

WHAT IS A SEXUALLY HEALTHY ADOLESCENT?

After reading the above information, you may feel skeptical that any teen could ever be "healthy." In conclusion, let's take a look at the qualities and characteristics of a sexually healthy adolescent.

A sexually healthy adolescent:

+ Respects and appreciates his or her own body
+ Expresses love and intimacy in appropriate ways
+ Avoids exploitive relationships
+ Communicates effectively with family and friends
+ Takes responsibility for his or her own behavior

✦ Asks questions of parents and other adults regarding sexual issues
✦ Enjoys sexual feelings without necessarily acting upon them
✦ Assertively communicates and negotiates sexual limits
✦ Understands the consequences of sexual activity
✦ Communicates desires not to engage in sexual activity and accepts refusals respectfully
✦ Is in the process of deciding what is personally "right" and acts in accordance with these values
✦ Demonstrates tolerance for people with different values
✦ Talks with a partner about sexual activity before it occurs, including limits, contraceptive and condom use, and meaning in the relationship
✦ Is aware of and understands the impact of media messages on thoughts, feelings, values, and behaviors related to sexuality
✦ Practices health-promoting behaviors, such as regular checkups, breast and testicular self-exams
✦ Interacts with both genders in appropriate and respectful ways
✦ Seeks further information about sexuality as needed

PARENTAL ISSUES: YOUR ADOLESCENCE

In order to have empathy and patience for your adolescent during the tumultuous teen years, you will need to remind yourself of the excitement, anxiety, fears, and embarrassment of your own adolescence. Spend some time remembering what it was like for you during those intense, important years.

✦

EXERCISE
Remembering Your Adolescence

Take some time to remember exactly how you felt when you were an adolescent; remember the feelings of rejection, your crushes, your first date. Remember how you felt about your parents during this time, the kind of questions you had about sexuality, and what you would have liked to have received from them in the way of sex education. Remember the struggles and conflicts you experienced and your difficulties with your parents and peers (especially around the issue of sexuality). Think about how you would have liked your parents to have handled conflicts with you.

✦

"GOING ALL THE WAY" FOR THE FIRST TIME

Whatever your experiences of sex were when you were a child, the first time you voluntarily decided to have sexual intercourse with someone of your choosing was no doubt a tremendously significant event in your life. This occurs for most of us when we are adolescents.

Take some time to think about your first experience. Remember the fears, the misconceptions, the feelings before and after the experience.

+ What was your motivation for having sex the first time?
+ What did you imagine it would be like?
+ Were you disappointed or pleasantly surprised?
+ Were you afraid that your parents would find out?
+ What did you imagine their reaction would be?
+ How did you feel around your parents afterward?
+ Were you afraid of pregnancy?
+ Were you concerned about how it would affect your relationship with your lover?

Remembering what it was like to be an adolescent and your first experience with sexual intercourse will help you not only to have more empathy for your child, but will also point out any feelings you still carry that may color your relationship with your child.

Although we all survived adolescence, some of us did it more successfully than others. Many, many people still have horror stories to tell about their teenage years, and some feel so humiliated that they still don't want to talk about it. Unfortunately, all too often our image of ourself as an adolescent seems to stick with us throughout adulthood, no matter how attractive or successful we become as adults. For some people, this old self-image is like an albatross around their neck, influencing their sexuality in a number of ways—from whether they feel sexually desirable to questions about their sexual identity.

Don't let your own negative experiences with sex as an adolescent make you so bitter, angry, or afraid that you project those feelings onto your child. Do the best you can to prepare her or him for the complexities of sexuality, and then let your teen experience her or his own feelings and even make her or his own mistakes.

Clearly, the sexual events in our lives have had a tremendous effect on us. Continue your own sex history into the present time. When you have finished, take a look at where you are today. Do you have a satisfactory sexual relationship? Do you think your partner is satisfied with your sexual relationship? Do you talk about your sexual relationship with your partner? Are you monogamous, or has one of you had an affair? Will your partner help in educating your child in a healthy way? Do you trust him or her to do that?

Adolescence can be an exciting and frightening time for both you and your teenager. Your role as a parent during this time is to make certain that your child learns all he or she can about his or her sexual feelings, sexual development, and sexual safety without scaring the child so much that sex becomes something to be feared instead of something to look forward to and enjoy.

While it is understandable for you to be frightened given the unhealthy sexual world we live in, work hard not to pass on your fears to your child. Instead, teach your teen safety, responsibility, and respect for his or her body. This will go a lot further than scare tactics, which will more than likely cause him or her to rebel. Remember that adolescence is a time when your child needs to assert her or his independence. Teach your teen all you can, and then begin to let her or him go. Trust that even though he or she will soon no longer be dependent on you, your child will take all your many lessons and your positive example with them.

14

♦

Special Problems of Adolescence

A dolescence is already a difficult time for teens, but for some it is particularly troublesome. In this chapter I will discuss special problems that many adolescents and their families are faced with, including:

✦ Sexual acting out
✦ Sexually active single parents as role models
✦ Helping your teen survive a broken heart
✦ Teens who become pregnant or are responsible for a pregnancy
✦ Teens who think they are homosexual

SEXUAL ACTING OUT

Many adolescents act out sexually (becoming sexual at too early an age, being sexually promiscuous, flaunting their sexual involvement) and go against their parents' values either as a way of communicating another need (such as a need for attention or acceptance), as a symptom of a problem (such as low self-esteem), or as a way of getting back at a parent (using sex as a battleground). Teens often act out sexually in response to their parents' getting divorced or remarried. And those teens who were sexually abused as children will often exhibit problems with their sexual identity, promiscuity, or having an attraction to "illicit" sexual activities such as pornography and prostitution.

If your teen is acting out sexually, it will do no good for you to rant and rave about his or her behavior. You must see this sexual acting out as a cry for help, not as a sign that he or she is a "bad" kid. Even if you suspect that he or she is involved in acting-out behavior as a way of getting a rise out of you or as a way to get you back for something you've done, your teenager is still crying out for help. No child chooses to act out sexually unless he or she is already in deep trouble.

While our first sexual encounters have a tremendous effect of our self-esteem, the reverse is also true. Our first sexual encounters will almost always reflect whatever fears, confusion, and self-esteem problems already exist within us. For instance, a young girl who feels inadequate and unattractive may hope to find approval through sexual acting out, but finds only disappointment and shame. A young man who is insecure and afraid concerning his own abilities may seek out sexual experiences, but his fear will permeate these experiences, coloring them in such a way as to make him feel even more insecure.

In addition, sometimes our first sexual experiences are primarily aimed at "getting back" at our parents or resisting the control of our parents, and have little to do with our being ready for sex. In these cases, the first experiences are not filled with love, connection, or nurturing, but rather anger, hurt, and confusion.

If your teen is sexually acting out, try sitting down and talking to her or him in a quiet, nonjudgmental way about her or his behavior. Let your child know that you are very concerned about his or her behavior and that you want to know how you can help. Ask if your child knows why he or she is involved in this behavior, what it provides in terms of a payback. The chances are high that she or he will not know or will not be willing to talk to you about it even if she or he does, but at least give it a try.

Because sexual acting out is so often a symptom of childhood sexual abuse, ask your teen if he or she was ever sexually molested. And be prepared for the answer. Assure your child that she or he can trust you and that you will believe her or him, no matter who the abuser was. If you get nowhere with this, then you will need to get some professional help.

Tell your teen that you would like it if he or she would agree to counseling. He or she may balk at the idea or even refuse. It is usually best not to try to force an adolescent into therapy, so if he or she refuses, don't push. Ask your child, as a favor to you, if he or she would agree to three sessions. Most teens are willing to at least try counseling if they don't feel forced and if it is time-limited. A lot can happen in three sessions if the counselor is good and if your teen is willing to open up. Your child may develop such a good connection with the counselor that he or she wants to continue.

If your teen refuses to attend the three sessions, ask if she or he would be willing to enter into family therapy. Some teens who are unwilling to enter individual therapy because they feel put on the spot, or because they fear the unknown, will agree to having the entire family seek help. If your teen agrees, this could also be a clue that the cause of the problem can be found in the family dynamics. Family therapy may be just the forum your teen needs to open up and discuss what is bothering her or him.

Spend some time assessing what part you may have in your teen's sexual acting-out behavior. For example, it is common for teens to act out sexually against overly rigid parental rules such as not allowing any dating or refusing to let the teenager wear makeup. Reevaluate family rules and family interactions to see if there is something that needs to be changed. Ask your teen what he or she would change in the family, and then *listen* to his or her suggestions without getting defensive. See if what your child is saying makes sense and if his or her suggestions can be implemented. Above all, constantly remind yourself that his or her sexual acting out is a symptom of a deeper problem.

SEXUALLY ACTIVE SINGLE PARENTS AS ROLE MODELS

It is difficult to balance raising a teen and having a personal sex life when you are a single parent. Married couples can go into their bedroom and close the door, but it is a great deal more complicated for a single parent. Every time you stay over at someone's house or have someone spend the night at yours, you are making a statement about sex. This is likely to make your child think "Hey, you're having sex with others, and you're not married to them, why can't I? How come I'm supposed to wait until I'm married, and you're not?"

Those parents who encourage their teens to wait until marriage often find that they have to defend their own actions, as Carl did:

I told my son, I'm older and more experienced. I can make better judgments and am more capable of dealing with any possible consequences.

Other parents do not set themselves up to look like hypocrites by demanding abstinence until marriage. They assume their teen will probably have sex before marriage, and they feel they themselves have a right to have sex outside of marriage. This is what Christine told her teenage daughter, who ironically was criticizing her for having sex outside of marriage:

Look, I've always told you that you have a right to your sexual feelings and that I didn't expect you to remain a virgin until marriage. I've just asked you to be careful whom you choose as a partner and to be sure that you are emotionally ready for sex. I'm an adult woman who has been married before and is used to having a sexual relationship with a man. But I don't want to make the mistake of marrying a man just because I am sexually attracted to him, and I wouldn't want you to either.

Some people will feel that the two parents in the above examples are actually being good role models because they are being honest instead of sneaking around and because they are being realistic for the present times. Others will feel that no matter what they tell their teens, they are being poor role models.

If you feel that you are being a poor role model because you are not practicing what you preach, it may help you to know that most single parents have ongoing relationships and/or sexual encounters. (According to researcher Morton Hunt, five out of six people become sexually active within the first year of separation.) You can have a sex life and still appear to be responsible and stable to your children. For example, unless you believe a relationship is going to last for some time, it is best not to spend the night together at your home if your children are there. You probably don't want to model to your child that it is okay to have sex with people you don't know very well or care little about.

In addition, some teens worry about their parent's getting a "bad reputation," are apprehensive about their parent's being "used," or being hurt. They want their parent to be happy, and they don't object to their parent trying to find someone new to love; it is the nomadic character of sexual relationships that seems to bother teens the most.

Once you have established an ongoing relationship and your child has had ample time to get to know your new partner, it will be easier for her or him to accept both the new person in your life and the fact that you are being sexual with one another. Most single parents have found that it is best to be honest about their sexual relationship instead of sneaking around or pretending that they are having a platonic relationship. They realize their teen is smart enough to figure out that Jeff or Susan doesn't spend the whole night on the couch.

Remember that the best way for children to learn about

healthy sexuality is by observing a loving, caring relationship at home. This does not necessarily mean that you have to be married to your partner to set an example of healthy communication, affection, and honesty. On the other hand, if you are involved in an unhealthy relationship where your child witnesses disrespect, dishonesty, sexual manipulation, or hears crude sexual language or innuendos, he or she will be learning negative messages about sex, whether you are married to your partner or not.

HELPING YOUR TEEN SURVIVE A BROKEN HEART

When you see your son or daughter feeling miserable over someone's breaking up with him or her, you will want to give comfort, try to cheer your child up, let her or him know that this too will pass. But often, instead of being open to your efforts, your teen will isolate her or himself from you and everyone else close to her or him, or because your teen is feeling rejected, take the anger and hurt out on you. But just because your teen tells you he or she doesn't need help, doesn't make it so. In reality, your teen can use all the help you can give. At the very least, he or she needs assurance that you will be there when he or she needs you to listen. And if your teen seems open to it, you can offer some strategies for "getting over" the relationship by following these suggestions:

+ Reassure your teen that what he or she is going through is normal. Educate your teen about the five basic stages of mourning: denial (when you can't believe it's over), anger, depression, bargaining (when you think you can do something to get back together), and finally, acceptance.
+ Encourage your teen to feel her or his sadness and pain, to go ahead and cry as much as she or he needs to.
+ Encourage your child not to feel inadequate, blame him or herself, obsess about the "if onlys," or play the breaking-up scene over and over in his or her mind.

- ✦ Encourage your teen to put his or her thoughts down on paper—the anger, pain, guilt—as a way of releasing his or her feelings and getting a better perspective.
- ✦ Encourage your child to release her or his anger in safe and constructive ways—hit the bed with a tennis racket, use a pillow to scream into, play tennis, racquetball, or volleyball and pretend the ball is the "ex."
- ✦ Encourage him or her to keep up with schoolwork and extracurricular activities. Let your teen know that it helps to keep your outer world in order when your inner world is in chaos.

TEENS WHO BECOME PREGNANT OR ARE RESPONSIBLE FOR A PREGNANCY

Your first reaction to hearing the news that your daughter is pregnant or your son is responsible for a pregnancy will probably be denial: "Are you sure?" "How do you know?" "That's not possible, you are too young."

Next, you may feel overwhelmed with anger and disappointment: "How could you?" "I can't believe you're telling me this after all the talks we had." "Well, now you've done it, you've ruined your life." Hopefully you can keep these kinds of thoughts to yourself; or, after an initial outburst, collect yourself and talk to your teen using "I" statements that focus on your feelings instead of on her or his character: "I'm very upset and very disappointed in you." "I find it difficult to believe that you could allow this to happen." "I hoped you would use better judgment."

Although you may feel devastated by the news, don't assassinate your child's character and make him or her feel any worse than he or she already does. Even though you may feel like it at the time, your child's life is not over, and you want to encourage her or him to make more mature decisions and to act more responsibly in the future, not make your child feel so ashamed that she or he will feel hopeless. Share how you feel, but do what you can to keep his or her self-esteem intact.

In the case of a daughter's pregnancy, since you do not have the luxury of time, you will immediately need to help her explore her options. As much as possible, encourage your daughter to make the decision herself by weighing the advantages and disadvantages of each option: marriage; abortion; having the baby and putting it up for adoption; having the baby and then placing the baby in a foster home where your daughter and the baby's father could visit the child until such time as they (or he or she) are ready to keep the child; having the child and keeping her home where you, the grandparents, could take over much of the child care.

Act as a guide and resource person, but try to keep your opinions to yourself. Ultimately, your daughter must take responsibility for her choice. Otherwise, she will blame you later on for trying to influence her too much or for not allowing her to do what she felt was right. You can help her to gain clarity about the situation by asking her the following questions:

+ How does your boyfriend feel about the pregnancy? If you decide to keep the baby, will he help you with hospital costs? Can he help support the child?
+ If you decide to keep the baby, have you thought about how you will react to your friends seeing you pregnant? What is the policy of your school about pregnant students?
+ Since you feel you want to give the baby up for adoption, have you thought about how you will feel giving up your baby? How do you think you will feel knowing all your life that you have a child out there somewhere who doesn't know you?
+ Have you considered how you will feel about getting an abortion? Do you think you will one day regret your decision?

Try to help your daughter make her decision based on what is best for the baby as well as what will be best for her. Let her know that you will support her decision whatever it is . . . to help her in any way that you can. One way of doing this is to make sure she is better informed about birth control and to reeducate her about the responsibility of sex.

Even though she is still a child in many ways and her judgment may not be very good, it is her body, and she needs to be the one who ultimately makes this important decision (one that will stay with her all her life). If she simply cannot make up her mind, suggest she receive psychological counseling. You can also suggest she visit your local Planned Parenthood office for a consultation.

Parents of sons who have impregnated girls need basically to follow the same suggestions as given above. Share your distress and disappointment with him without making him feel terrible about himself; hold him responsible for what he has done; insist that he participate in the many decisions that need to be made; but let him know that you are behind him all the way and that he still has a future in which he can act responsibly and achieve success. It is also important that you let your son know that he has rights. Current law now dictates that the father has a right to keep the child himself if the mother decides to have the child adopted.

TEENS WHO THINK THEY ARE HOMOSEXUAL

What do you do if your teenager comes to you and tells you he's gay or she's lesbian? First of all, try not to panic. Make sure you don't say anything you can never take back. It is already so difficult for young people to talk to their parents about their fears and feelings about homosexuality—don't make it any harder than it has to be. Most gay men and lesbian women report that the most difficult part of realizing they are homosexual isn't coming to terms with themselves, but telling their parents. And there is good reason for their trepidation. Most parents feel as though they have been hit by a Mack truck when they hear their child say, "I'm gay." It will help if you realize that your child isn't doing anything "to you" (as in

"How could you do this to me?"). They are doing what is right for themselves.

It will also help if you remind yourself just how much courage it took for your lesbian daughter or gay son to come forward and tell the family. She or he is showing a great deal of trust by confiding in you and by acknowledging her or his need for your acceptance.

Most parents would hope that they could suppress their misgivings and react with loving acceptance. But even the most liberal, tolerant parents, no matter how nonjudgmental and accepting of homosexuality for others, may have a difficult time when it comes to discovering that their own child is homosexual. The initial reaction is most commonly shock, followed by the fear that their child will contract AIDS, and grief and mourning for what they perceive as all the lost dreams of wedding and grandchildren. Then many parents are overcome with guilt ("Where did I go wrong?") and shame ("How could my child do this thing?").

It is perfectly okay to share your honest feelings with your teenager as long as you don't put her or him down and as long as you use "I" statements. For example, it is appropriate that you share your shock or even disappointment: "I can't believe it. You've got to be kidding." "I'm shocked. I had no idea." "I feel so disappointed." "I fear for the life you have chosen." Your teenager is far more likely to trust you if you are honest with how you are feeling instead of pretending to feel something you are not.

Because homosexuality still provokes hostility and discrimination from others, parents cannot help but view this news as their child entering adulthood with one strike against him or her. It is also perfectly normal to worry about what others "will think." Chances are that many friends and relatives will be shocked, and some may be critical or outright rejecting. Added to your fear that your child will be rejected, isolated, and face prejudice is the deadly reality of AIDS. It is absolutely horrifying to imagine your child contracting this dreaded disease.

At any rate, it's better for your child and for you that he or she has brought the subject out in the open rather than constantly worrying about being "found out" and living a life in which you are kept in the dark or from which you are excluded. Growing up homosexual and pretending to be heterosexual is a distorted, absurd way of living. The lying and deceiving is damaging to the child and to the family. It often continues into adulthood with the person trying to conform to society's expectations by marrying and then establishing a double life.

WHAT TO DO AND WHAT NOT TO DO

It is vitally important that you increase your understanding about homosexuality. Learn all you can about homosexuality from books, videos, courses, and discussion groups. If you have trouble locating resources, contact your local gay community services and ask what they have to offer parents.

Don't waste energy and time in trying to figure out what you did wrong. The chances are very high that you did nothing to cause your child's homosexuality. We still know very little about what actually causes homosexuality, whether it is something a child is born with or something that develops because of the child's environment and life experiences. It would seem, from all indications, that perhaps some people are born homosexual, some become homosexual because of trauma such as child sexual abuse or rape, and some choose to be homosexual because of their political beliefs. The point here is that homosexuality is not a disease that you should try to find the cause or cure for. It is a sexual orientation, nothing more and nothing less.

Different is a good word to describe homosexuality because it does not imply sickness. Homosexuality is not an illness, as changes in psychiatric diagnoses now indicate. Homosexuals are neither sick nor crazy. They are not suffering from a psychological state that can be "cured" by therapy in the way that therapy can alleviate anxiety or depression. It is no longer believed that homosexuality is caused by any one thing. Homosexuals exist in every culture and society. Many cultures find homosexuality acceptable. Our culture has frowned on it.

Another, more difficult concept is that homosexuality is not generally a matter of will. In the same way that a heterosexual cannot generally "will" himself or herself to practice homosexuality as a permanent lifestyle, a homosexual cannot "will" himself or herself to practice heterosexuality.

Some of my clients have told me that when they think back, they have known they were different since the age of five. Others have reported a gradually developing realization of their sexuality. Many have resisted that change vigorously. Many are deeply unhappy that they are homosexual, and many are proud of their sexuality and regard it as a declaration of individual freedom to be what they are.

Don't try to change your child to heterosexuality. While our first reaction to anything unpleasant is usually denial ("You're so young, how could you know?" "Maybe this is just a phase you're going through." "Maybe you'll change your mind."), you owe it to your child to work on accepting her or him the way the child is instead of trying to change her or him.

Change is rare—not totally impossible, but infrequent. Even those who resent their homosexuality and would prefer the straight life find it difficult to live that way. Many people have gone into therapy looking for help to make this change, but have ended their therapy accepting themselves.

There is always the remote possibility that your child is using homosexuality as a way to be different from you, to get your attention, or to test your capacity to accept him or her. If this is the case, pressuring him or her to change will only cause the child to hold tighter to his or her behavior.

No matter how you feel about your child's homosexuality, don't try to change or punish her or him by casting the child out of the family. In almost all cases, this tactic has failed. It does not help the child and, in the long run, becomes inordinately painful for the parents. If you banish your child, siblings may miss her or him terribly and blame you. Other relatives may have more tolerance and may secretly continue their relationship, and this may in turn cause a separation between them and you.

Be aware, though, that maintaining the relationship may not be easy. You may be asked to meet your child's lover, to invite him or her to your home, or to be a guest at the couple's home. Although that may be difficult, it is amazing how your feelings can change when you contemplate losing your child instead. In time, as you get to know your child's lover and observe their relationship (especially if it is a positive one), you will become more and more comfortable.

It would be most helpful to both you and your child if you work toward getting to the place where you care more about the *quality* of your child's relationships rather than the *kind* of relationships he or she has. In addition, it is important to realize that we experience a sense of total well-being when all aspects of ourselves fit together—physical, emotional, and spiritual. This phenomenon is not present for people who have to pretend to be something they are not, or who fantasize about someone of the same sex while being expected to be attracted to someone of the opposite sex.

Every family reacts differently. Some families go into mourning over the "loss" of their child, some parents suffer severe depression, some parents get angry and reject their child completely. And some families accept their child's companion as they would accept husband or wife.

A homosexual relationship can be one of lasting love, the same as any heterosexual relationship. Gay people have similar fights and similar differences.

Maintain the same values with your homosexual child that you have previously shown. Encourage responsibility—to him or herself and his or her associates. Encourage healthy limit-setting, and model this by setting your own limits.

And last but not least, while you don't want to try to make your teen into something he or she is not or to discount his or her sexual preference as a "passing phase," you may want to encourage your child not to jump to conclusions and to keep his or her options open. Most experts on the subject feel that deciding during early adolescence that one is definitely and permanently homosexual may be premature. We know that adolescents go through many changes as they mature. Your child may find he or she feels differently later on about exclusive preference, or any desire at all, for partners of the same sex. While it is true that by late adolescence most people are clear about their sexual orientation, there are significant numbers of young people whose sexual orientation isn't clearly defined until later in life.

Suggest that your teen consider seeing a counselor, not in order to be "cured" of homosexuality, but to help her or him sort out feelings and to enhance a positive sense of self-esteem. It would be a rare adolescent who doesn't have some problems adjusting to the realization that she or he is or could be homosexual in a heterosexual world. Make sure you choose the therapist carefully, one who specializes in and understands sexual orientation. If your teen is reluctant to seek counseling, don't push it. By all means do not give her or him the message that there is something wrong with her or him. Let your child know that you support her or his decision either way.

I recommend family therapy as well as individual treatment for several reasons. First of all, family therapy eliminates the notion that the homosexual family member is "the sick one," helps all members of the family to adjust, and helps maintain the family as a unit.

There are many organizations and sources of counseling and services available to your child. They will direct her or him to groups that will provide peer support to counter the isolation that these young people experience.

There are also many resources now available for parents as well. I strongly recommend P-Flag, a support group for parents of homosexuals. Please refer to Appendix I.

The special problems addressed in this chapter—sexual acting out, being a sexually active single parent, helping your teen overcome a broken heart, teen pregnancy, your teen's concerns about homosexuality—can make adolescence, an already difficult period of time, even more trying. But as you've read, these are problems that can be handled and handled well if you and your teen talk to one another, listen to one another, and work together.

Parental Issues: Your Special Problems During Adolescence

It is highly likely that when you were a teen you too suffered from one or more of the special problems we have discussed in this chapter. Unfortunately, these problems may be the very ones your teen will experience, since history does tend to repeat itself. Sometimes it happens as a kind of self-fulfilling prophecy. For example, you are so afraid your teen will get pregnant as you did that you set the scene for it to happen. Parents do this in many ways, including constantly nagging at the teen about it, accusing her or him of it, or assuming it's going to happen.

One way to avoid this is for you to complete your unfinished business about the situation. This may involve entering therapy or joining a support group, or you may be able to process it by any of the following ways:

✦ Talk to your spouse or a good friend about it. Allow yourself to feel all the pent-up emotions that you may have held in all this time.

✦ Write about the situation, again expressing all your repressed and suppressed emotions.

✦ Do some anger release work such as hitting a pillow, talking out loud to an imaginary person (such as your parent, the boy who made you pregnant and abandoned you, the girl who broke your heart, the man who raped you), or writing a letter to this person that you may or may not choose to send expressing all your anger and pain.

◆

EXERCISE

If you did experience one of the special problems listed in this chapter, answer the following questions:

1. Why do you think this problem occurred?
2. Could this problem have been avoided? If so, how?
3. How would you have preferred your parents to have handled the problem?

◆

Your answers to these questions may be more beneficial than any of the advice I've shared with you and may be just the ammunition you need to help you handle these special problems if they do occur with your teen.

15

Final Thoughts

There is a lot more to healthy sexuality than the sex act itself. Healthy sexual relationships also involve intimacy, tenderness, trust, and sensuality. They involve being able to ask for what you want sexually, being able to give honest feedback, and being able to seek out appropriate partners.

Sexual contact is always more fulfilling in the context of openness, tenderness, and sensitivity to the needs of the other person. When sexual release comes in the context of trust, commitment, and safety, its pleasures take on heightened meaning.

And ultimately, sex is the most exciting when it is combined with love. Love that has any depth means involvement. True love is about loving and supporting one another, not trying to change one another, but accepting one another the way you are. Parents must model trust and intimacy for their children and teens, teach and model good communication skills, and continually focus on raising their child's self-esteem.

THE FEAR OF INTIMACY

Intimate sex—sex that is meant as an expression of love or affection, as a way for two people who care for one another to connect in a meaningful way—involves being willing and able to be open and vulnerable, to trust another person, to be desirous of pleasing another person, and at the same time to be willing to express one's own needs.

When you become intimate with someone, you are letting yourself really be seen and known. That is why intimacy can be so frightening to most of us. The vulnerability and openness of an intimate relationship can feel deeply threatening because when we open ourselves up to another, that person has the ability to hurt us emotionally the way no one else can.

As your teenager or young adult begins to establish intimacy with a partner, he or she may feel unsafe and respond by withdrawing or building barriers between him or herself and his or her sexual partner, or by sabotaging the relationship as Ted did:

> Every time I get really close to my girlfriend, I end up doing something to destroy our closeness. I pick a fight, or get critical of her, and then we break up for a while. We eventually get back together, but I'm afraid that one day she won't come back to me. I don't know why I do this—it seems I can't help myself.

Even though your teen may consciously want to have a close, intimate relationship, something in his or her subconscious can set out to destroy the relationship whenever he or she feels they are getting too close. We sometimes unconsciously arrange our lives so that we're on a kind of roller coaster, running from involvement and then breaking up, so that we feel totally independent. Then we climb back on the roller coaster and begin all over again.

Another way of avoiding intimacy is to distance ourselves sexually, thinking of sex as an activity rather than as a deep sharing of our innermost selves. Men tend to do this more than women, but both sexes are capable of it. Years ago, it used to be believed that males were less interested in and had less need for intimacy, but studies have shown this not to be true. Both men and women need and want intimacy; it is equally important for happiness to both sexes.

Still another way of dealing with a fear of intimacy is to allow ourselves to share intimately while we're being sexual, but avoid vulnerability in our day-to-day life with our partner.

Or, we may find a certain level of intimacy comfortable in our sexual relationship, but tend to panic when the relationship begins to deepen and grow. This happens most often when the intimacy of sexuality touches early childhood wounds.

In fact, our fear of intimacy probably begins in our childhood. Anxiety about intimacy can usually be traced to a faulty relationship with parents or to childhood abuse.

While adolescence is a time for teens to experiment and explore a variety of relationships, it is also a time when most teens fall in love for the first time and have sex for the first time. It is a time when they begin to experience emotional and sexual intimacy with a partner. If you notice that your teen is continually breaking up and then making up with her boyfriend or his girlfriend or continually fighting with her or his partner, he or she may be having problems with intimacy.

THE RISKS OF INTIMACY

Learning to be intimate in a sexual relationship takes time, and it requires being willing to take risks. Obviously, these risks should be taken slowly and carefully and even systematically— not haphazardly. This means taking a sexual or emotional risk when it is appropriate to how vulnerable it makes you feel at that stage of the relationship. Intimacy is often established one step at a time by taking a risk, then stepping back and giving yourself some time before you take another.

Encourage your teen to begin with a small risk that doesn't have an enormous consequence if it doesn't work out. If it does work out, then he or she can move on to a bigger risk. Encourage your teen continually to reassess the relationship and what is happening to him or her all along the way and to keep asking himself or herself if he or she is being honest with himself or herself and with the partner, both sexually and emotionally.

Explain to your teen that if she or he begins to hide her or his feelings from the partner, then there is surely a problem in the relationship. It is essential to intimacy that we be able to express our feelings and that we be able to trust that our partner will honor those feelings. If your teen has begun to hide his or her feelings, he or she should ask himself or herself whether the relationship still feels equal, mutual, and reciprocal (whether one has more power than the other in the relationship, and whether he or she and the partner are giving and receiving at similar levels). Suggest that your teen ask himself or herself whether the level of trust is growing or whether the two of them are distancing and withdrawing.

Not every sexual relationship has the capacity for intimacy. Suggest that your teen ask the following questions concerning a sexual partner to help her or him determine whether it is wise to take the risk of true intimacy:

- ✦ Do I truly respect this person, and does he or she seem to respect me?
- ✦ Is this a person I can communicate openly with, and does he or she seem able to communicate openly with me?
- ✦ Am I able to be honest with this person, or am I lying, covering up, or putting up a facade?
- ✦ Do I believe this person is able to be honest with me?
- ✦ Do I feel safe enough to show my real feelings with this person?
- ✦ Are we both able to compromise with one another?
- ✦ Do we work through conflicts well?
- ✦ Do we both take responsibility for the problems of the relationship, or does one of us continually blame the other?
- ✦ Can I talk to this person about my childhood experiences, no matter how embarrassing they are?
- ✦ Can I talk to this person about my former relationships?
- ✦ Am I willing to talk about how I feel my past is affecting our relationship, and is my partner willing to do the same?
- ✦ Is it possible for me to be myself in this relationship?
- ✦ Is there room for me to grow and change in this relationship?

If his or her relationship continues to deepen and to develop, your teen can then take greater risks that require still more vulnerability. By carefully and systematically taking risks one step at a time in a relationship, and then sitting back to assess the level of trust and openness, he or she can create a healthy, conscious relationship instead of one driven by fear, compulsion, or unfulfilled childhood needs.

COMMUNICATING OPENLY ABOUT SEX

You've heard this before—good communication between partners is as essential to sexual pleasure (and to good sex in general) as is any particular technique. A survey conducted by Philip and Lorna Sarrel, sex therapists at Yale University, concluded that the ability to share thoughts and feelings about sex with your partner is the single most important factor in a good sexual relationship.

Teach your teen that in an established relationship it is important that you tell your partner what you need in order to feel loved, and it is also important that you listen to what your partner says he or she needs. Teach your teen that it is equally important to open up the communication early in a new relationship. Because of the lack of familiarity with each other, it makes it even more important to share specific information early on. Also, letting your partner know early in the relationship what you like and don't like sexually helps to prevent negative patterns from developing.

In new relationships, people make love to their new partner by doing what turns themselves on, by doing what pleased a previous partner, or by doing what they have read women or men like. During the "honeymoon period" in a new relationship, everything tends to feel good, but people become more discriminating as time goes by. At that point, if you don't let your partner know what turns you on or off, you will only reinforce the belief that what is being done is okay, thus encouraging your partner to continue as before.

Teach your teen that he or she has the right to ask for what he or she wants with a sexual partner. Many people have the belief that their partner should be sensitive enough to their needs to know automatically what they want without their having to ask for it. How often have you heard someone say, "If I have to ask for it, I don't want it." When you think about this, it seems rather silly, doesn't it? Don't allow this kind of misguided thinking to get in your teen's way of receiving the kind of touches and stimulation that he or she really desires. Tell your teen that no one is a mind reader, and no matter how well his or her partner knows them, there is really no way he or she can know what they want sexually at any given time.

Some people are afraid to ask for what they want sexually for fear of being rejected. If they are able to ask at all, they couch their requests in subtle language, hoping their wishes will be understood, but protecting themselves in case they're not. Unfortunately, the fear of not getting their wishes can create a self-fulfilling prophecy. If you don't ask for what you want directly, your partner may never know what you want. And if you interpret not getting what you want as an indication that you were right not to ask because you wouldn't have gotten what you wanted anyway, then you won't make your needs known the next time either. Although it is difficult, being vulnerable with your partner by openly communicating your sexual preferences is an excellent way of building trust in your partner.

People who love each other want to please each other, but they often do not know how. Men in particular often report that they wish their partners would be more clear when they communicate their needs so they wouldn't have to fumble around trying to figure out her wishes. By not being specific enough with her or his partner about her or his sexual preferences, your teen is not only depriving her or himself of sexual pleasure, but depriving the partner of the pleasure of pleasing her or him.

HOW SELF-ESTEEM AFFECTS SEXUALITY

When I was on a book tour for my last book, *Raising Your Sexual Self-Esteem*, the question I was asked most often was, "How can I make sure that I don't pass on my sexual problems, fears, and hang-ups to my children? How can we raise our children to have high sexual self-esteem?" I was happy to tell my audiences that I was going to address this issue in my next book, *Beyond the Birds and the Bees*.

What exactly is sexual self-esteem? Put simply, our sexual self-esteem is a measure of how we feel about ourselves sexually. The level of our sexual self-esteem determines just how sexually attractive we feel we are to others, how confident we feel about our sexuality, how responsive we are sexually, and how free we are to express our sexual feelings. It includes how we feel about our ability to satisfy our sexual partners, how we feel about our bodies, and how "normal" we feel we are regarding our sex drive, our sexual orientation, and our ability to perform sexually.

No matter how good your child's sex education classes are, no matter how informed your child is about sex through books and the media, parents are the only ones who can teach their children the most significant lessons about sex they will ever need to know, namely:

- ✦ That sexual feelings and reactions including masturbation and sexual fantasies are all normal and healthy.
- ✦ That we should never allow ourselves to be coerced or manipulated into doing *anything* sexually that we do not have the interest, curiosity, or desire for.
- ✦ That we should love and respect our body.
- ✦ That we should always choose partners who compliment and appreciate our body, who accept us the way we are, and who respect our limits.

✦ That we should always have equal relationships.
✦ That we should never engage in esteem-robbing activities.

These are the components of high sexual self-esteem.

Throughout the book you may have noticed that I have often referred to self-esteem. A child with high self-esteem is far more likely to be a sexually healthy child and one who will grow up to have a fulfilling sex life.

Your child's sexuality is immensely affected by how high or low his or her self-esteem is. Low self-esteem can affect our sexuality in a number of ways. If we don't feel good about ourselves, we may avoid sexual relationships because we are afraid of intimacy. We may be afraid of allowing another person to get too close to us and thus to find out who we "really" are.

Or, perhaps we have sexual relationships, but tend to hold back from experiencing pleasure either because we don't think we deserve it or because it makes us feel guilty. Similarly, we may avoid masturbation because it makes us feel guilty, or we believe we are undeserving of pleasure or that physical pleasure is not worth the time or energy.

Or, we may become involved with one unhappy and exploitive sexual affair after another, either because we are so uncertain of our worth that we feel driven constantly to prove our sexual attractiveness or prowess, or because we believe we do not deserve to be treated well.

When our self-esteem is low, we tend to get involved with sexual partners and sexual practices that reflect and reinforce our poor image of ourselves, leaving us with less self-esteem than we had before. Promiscuity, prostitution, sadomasochism, and sexual addiction are all manifestations of low self-esteem and in turn perpetuate it by causing those involved to feel isolated and full of shame and humiliation.

If your child's self-esteem is low, if he or she has a poor opinion of himself or herself, chances are he or she is not going to feel physically and sexually attractive to others. He or she will not be as motivated either to initiate a new relationship or to initiate sexuality in an existing one. Or, uncertain of his or her worth, your child may feel driven constantly to prove his or her sexual attractiveness and prowess. He or she may tend to focus too much attention on his or her physical appearance and on "performing" rather than enjoying sex.

No matter what your child's body looks like, if he or she doesn't feel good about him or herself, if he or she doesn't basically like him or herself, he or she will feel unattractive. The less we like ourselves, the harder time we have understanding why someone else would like us or find us attractive. Low self-esteem thus causes us to focus too much attention on how our bodies look. We assume that it is our body that can either turn the other person on or turn the other person off, not recognizing that it is our entire person—our mind, our personality, and our very spirit that attracts another person.

When our self-esteem is high, we feel more attractive, desirable, and confident about our sexuality. We neither shy away from nor focus too much attention on sex. It becomes a natural part of our need to express ourselves and our caring for others. We choose sexual partners who treat us with respect and tenderness, and we get involved with sexual practices that are life-affirming and make us feel good about ourselves.

Keep all this in mind as you raise your child. Do all you can to enhance your child's self-esteem and to prevent things from occurring that will lower your child's self-esteem, such as childhood sexual abuse. Work especially hard to help your child feel good about his or her body because a good body image and high self-esteem go hand-in-hand.

Pay particular attention to how you talk to your child. Make sure you give lots of positive strokes for the way your child looks, his or her accomplishments, any positive changes in his or her attitude, and any acts of consideration and kindness.

Your child's self-esteem is particularly shaky during adolescence. Don't fall into the trap of relating to your teen only as a disciplinarian. Adolescents need lots and lots of positive feedback and encouragement. Work toward making the transition from parent/authority figure to the eventual role of friend/

confidant that you'll want to have when your child becomes an adult.

Last, but certainly not least, continue working on raising your own self-esteem and becoming a more sexually healthy adult. Remember that your job as a role model is as important as anything you teach your child.

How and Where to Get More Help

You may find that you need further information on a particular subject or concerning a troublesome issue. In the Bibliography are some suggestions for books to read on related topics. Sometimes parents need the kind of information that is more readily found by contacting a specific organization. Please refer to Appendix I for a list of organizations. In Appendix II you will find tips on how to locate a sex therapist.

Appendix I: Resources

SINGLE PARENTS

Parents Without Partners
(Concerns of single parents and their children)
Various chapters in U.S.
7910 Woodmont Avenue, Suite 1000
Bethesda, MD 20814
800-638-8078

CHILD SEXUAL ABUSE

To Report Child Abuse

Most states have a Child Abuse Hotline. To find yours, call information. Or, call the National Child Abuse Hotline:
800-422-4453

ECHO (Exploited Children's Help Organization)
1204 S. 3rd Street, Suite B
Louisville, KY 40203
502-637-8761

National Council on Child Abuse and Family Violence
1050 Connecticut Avenue, N.W.
Washington, D.C. 20036
202-429-6695

Prevention

National Crime Prevention Council
(Information and action kits for schools and parents)
1341 G Street, N.W., Suite 706
Washington, D.C. 20005
202-393-7141

SLAM (Society's League Against Molestation)
(Lobbies for strong legislation, offers "Cautious Kid" programs)
Various chapters in U.S.
303-755-5800

Support for Nonoffending and Offending Parents

Parents United
(Incest therapy and counseling)
Various chapters in U.S., based in San Jose, CA
408-280-5055

Parents Anonymous
800-421-0353

Help for Survivors of Childhood Sexual Abuse

VOICES (Victims of Incest Can Emerge Survivors) in Action, Inc.
(A national network of female and male survivors and prosurvivors—
supportive friends and family—that has local groups and contacts
throughout the U.S. Offers a free referral service that provides list-
ings of therapists, agencies, and self-help groups.)
P.O. Box 148309
Chicago, IL 60614
312-327-1500
In addition, two organizations help provide support groups nationwide for incest survivors:

Survivors of Incest Anonymous
P.O. Box 21817
Baltimore, MD 21222-6817
301-282-3400

Incest Survivors Anonymous
P.O. Box 5613
Long Beach, CA 90805-0613
213-428-5599

Preventing and Treating Rape

Rape crisis hotlines exist in all major cities. They are sometimes listed as "crisis hotlines."

Sources of Help for Sex Offenders

Parents United (see above)

Sex Addicts Anonymous
P.O. Box 3038
Minneapolis, MN 55403

Sexaholics Anonymous
P.O. Box 300
Simi Valley, CA 93062

Runaways

(Often running from sexual abuse at home)
The National Runaway Switchboard
800-621-4000
The National Runaway Hotline
800-231-6946

How to Report Sexual Harassment

Equal Employment Opportunity Commission
(Check the government section of your phone book)

Human Rights Commission
(Check your state capital for the number)

DISEASE PREVENTION AND BIRTH CONTROL

Sources of Information and/or Testing

(These services should always be confidential, but you may want to double-check to feel reassured. There are some state laws requiring the reporting of certain STDs to keep track for health purposes.)

Planned Parenthood has centers in most major cities in the U.S. and offers contraception and other services, depending on the center.

County health departments usually provide sites for testing and treatment of STDs.

AIDS prevention and AIDS support groups have sprung up in various locations and can refer you to testing sources. Check your phone book for AIDS agencies to get a referral.

Community services for AIDS
AIDS Foundation Hotlines

Gay community services

VD clinics

AIDS antibody testing is available through private physicians or public clinics.

Hotlines

National STD Hotline: 800-227-8922

National AIDS Hotline: 800-342-AIDS

National Herpes Hotline: 919-361-2120

For information on how to use a condom correctly, or to learn about high- and low-risk behaviors for any STD:

+ Call government-sponsored testing sites listed under your county's health department, or Planned Parenthood
+ Call the STD or the AIDS Hotline (above), or call your college health service

GAY, LESBIAN, BISEXUAL

PFLAG (Parents and Friends of Lesbians and Gays)
Box 24565
Los Angeles, CA 90024

The National Gay Task Force
80 Fifth Avenue
New York, NY 10011

Appendix II: How to Locate a Sex Therapist

Sometimes parents need to seek professional help for their children's problems. This is particularly true in the cases of sexual acting out, sexual-identity confusion, and sexual dysfunction.

- ✦ If you are comfortable doing so, ask friends, family members, or co-workers who have gone to a sex counselor whether they can recommend someone.
- ✦ Ask your family physician or clergyman for a recommendation.
- ✦ Write to one of the following groups and ask for a list of certified counselors and therapists in your area (there may be a nominal fee):

American Association of Sex Educators, Counselors, and Therapists (AASECT)
11 Dupont Circle, N.W., Suite 220
Washington, D.C. 20036

American Association for Marriage and Family Therapy (AAMFT)
1717 K Street, N.W., Suite 407
Washington, D.C. 20006

- ✦ Call your local Community Health Center and ask for recommendations, or call the nearest medical school or large hospital and ask if they have a sex dysfunction clinic.
- ✦ Look in the yellow pages of your telephone book under:

Clinical Social Workers
Marriage, Family, Child Counselors
Mental Health Services
Psychologists

Psychiatrists (may be listed under Physicians & Surgeons—
Medical-M.D.)

Sex therapists are usually not listed separately in the yellow
pages. Look under the above headings; if the individual specializes in sex counseling, it will be noted under his or her name.

If you suspect your child's sexual problems may include medical or physical factors, locate a sex therapist who works closely
with medical professionals, or a physician with special training
in sexual medicine.

Medical doctors are listed twice in the yellow pages under
Physicians, alphabetically, and by specialty. The doctors who
should know the most about AIDS are: a) infectious disease
specialists, b) urologists—who diagnose and treat disorders of
male genitalia and male and female urinary problems, c) gyne-
cologists—who diagnose and treat disorders of female genitalia
and reproductive organs.

✦ Call the nearest medical school, university, or large hospital,
and ask if they have a special clinic for diagnosing and treating
sexual problems (dysfunctions). If your town does not have
such a facility, most libraries have telephone directories of
nearby large cities.

Places to Call for Further Referrals

A number you can call for many kinds of referrals:

✦ National Self-Help Clearinghouse
212-642-2944

Bibliography and Recommended Reading

GENERAL

Brazelton, Berry. *On Becoming a Family: The Growth of Attachment.* New York: Dell, 1981.

Calderone, Mary, and Eric Johnson. *The Family Book About Sexuality.* New York: Bantam Books, 1983.

———, and J. W. Ramey. *Talking with Your Child About Sex: Questions and Answers for Children from Birth to Puberty.* New York: Random House, 1982.

Colao, Flora, and Tamar Hosansky. *Your Children Should Know.* Indianapolis and New York: Bobbs-Merrill, 1983.

Hechinger, Grace. *How to Raise a Street-Smart Child.* New York: Facts on File, 1984.

Scanzoni, L. D. *Sex Is a Parent Affair: A Responsible Guide for Teaching Your Children About Sex.* New York: Bantam Books, 1982.

FOR PARENTS OF TEENAGERS

Kolodny, Robert, et al. *How to Survive Your Adolescent's Adolescence.* New York: Little, Brown, 1984.

Oettinger, K. B., with E. C. Mooney. *Not My Daughter: Facing Up to Adolescent Pregnancy.* Englewood Cliffs, NJ: Prentice-Hall, 1979.

BOOKS FOR TEENS

Adams, Caren, et al. *No Is Not Enough: Helping Teens Avoid Sexual Assault.* San Luis Obispo, CA: Impact Publishers, 1984.

Gordon, Sol. *The Teenage Survival Book.* New York: Times Books, 1981.

————. *Facts About Sex For Today's Youth*. New York: Ed-U Press, 1983.

McCoy, K. *The Teenage Body Book*. New York: Wallaby, 1982.

FOR YOUNG ADULTS (AGES SIXTEEN AND UP)

Bell, R. *Changing Bodies, Changing Lives*. New York: Random House, 1981.

Comfort, A., and J. Comfort. *The Facts of Love: Living, Loving and Growing Up*. New York: Crown, 1980.

Johnson, Eric. *Love and Sex in Plain Language*, 4th ed. New York: Harper & Row, 1985.

Powell, Elizabeth. *Talking Back to Sexual Pressure*. Minnesota: Comp Care, 1991.

SEXUAL ABUSE

Engel, Beverly. *The Right to Innocence: Healing The Trauma of Childhood Sexual Abuse*. New York: Ivy Books, 1989.

————. *Families in Recovery: Working Together to Heal the Damage of Childhood Sexual Abuse*. Los Angeles: Lowell House, 1994.

Finkelhor, D., *Sexually Victimized Children*. New York: Free Press, 1979.

Lanning, Kenneth, and Ann Wolbert Burgess. "Child Pornography and Sex Rings." *FBI Law Enforcement Bulletin* (January 1984): 10–16.

Love, Patricia. *The Emotional Incest Syndrome*. New York: Bantam Books, 1991.

Sanford, Linda T. *The Silent Children: A Parents Guide to the Prevention of Child Sexual Abuse*. New York: Doubleday, 1980.

————. *Come Tell Me Right Away: A Positive Approach to Warning Children About Sexual Abuse*. Fayetteville, NY: Ed-U Press, 1982.

Wachter, Oralee. *No More Secrets for Me*. Boston: Little, Brown, 1983.

Wooden, Ken. *Child Lures: A Guide to Prevent Abduction*. Mascoutah, IL: Purina Ralston Co., 1984. (Also available from ABC-TV News.)

RAPE RECOVERY

Ledroy, Linda. *Recovering from Rape*. New York: Henry Holt & Co., 1986.

HOMOSEXUALITY

Austin, Al, and Keith Hefner, eds. *Growing Up Gay*. Ann Arbor: Youth Liberation Press, 1978.

Fairchild, Betty, and Nancy Hayward. *Now That You Know: What Every Parent Should Know About Homosexuality*. New York: Harcourt Brace Jovanovich, 1984.

SINGLE PARENTS

Adams, J. *Sex and the Single Parent*. New York: Coward, McCann & Geoghegan, 1978.

Weiss, R. S. *Going It Alone: The Family Life and Social Situation of the Single Parent*. New York: Basic Books, 1979.

BIRTH CONTROL

Hatcher, R. A., et al. *It's Your Choice: A Personal Guide to Birth Control Methods for Women—and Men Too*. New York: Irvington Publishers, 1982.

SEXUALLY TRANSMITTED DISEASES

Corsaro, M., and C. Korzeniowsky. *STD: A Commonsense Guide*. New York: St. Martin's Press, 1980.

Gordon, Sol. *Facts About STDs*. New York: Ed-U Press, 1983.

Lumiere, Richard, and Stephanie Cook. *Healthy Sex: And Keeping It That Way*. New York: Simon & Schuster, 1983.

The Complete Guide to Safe Sex. The Institute for Advanced Study of Human Sexuality. Beverly Hills: Specific Press, 1987.

SEXUAL SENSITIVITY

Barbach, L. *For Each Other: Sharing Sexual Intimacy.* New York: Doubleday Anchor, 1982.

For males:

Zilbergetld, B. *Male Sexuality: A Guide to Sexual Fulfillment.* Boston: Little, Brown, 1978.

For females:

Barbach, L. G. *For Yourself: The Fulfillment of Female Sexuality.* New York: Doubleday, 1975.

SELF-ESTEEM

Briggs, Dorothy Corkville. *Your Child's Self-Esteem.* New York: Dolphin Books, 1975.

Engel, Beverly. *Raising Your Sexual Self-Esteem.* New York: Fawcett Columbine, 1995.

VALUES

Eyre, Linda and Richard. *Teaching Your Children Values.* New York: Simon & Schuster, 1993.

Index